I0820154

HOW DO YOU Like It?

HOW DO YOU Like It?

A GUIDE *for* GETTING WHAT YOU WANT *(in Bed)*

DR. TARA SUWINYATTICHAIPORN

ABRAMS PRESS, NEW YORK

Published in 2025 by Abrams Press, an imprint of ABRAMS.

Library of Congress Control Number: 2025931665

ISBN: 978-1-4197-7643-4
eISBN: 979-8-88707-385-9

Printed and bound in the United States
10 9 8 7 6 5 4 3 2 1

ABRAMS The Art of Books
195 Broadway, New York, NY 10007
abramsbooks.com

ABRAMS is represented in the UK and Europe by
Abrams & Chronicle Books, 1 West Smithfield, London EC1A 9JU
and Média-Participations, 57 rue Gaston Tessier, 75166 Paris, France.
abramsandchronicle.co.uk | media-participations.com
info@abramsandchronicle.co.uk

To all the sex-positive icons before me whose works were necessary milestones to move sex positivity forward in this millennium.

Contents

Introduction: Become Your Own Sexpert

Sex isn't just about sex.
Sex is about everything else.

It's 8 a.m. on a Monday, and it's sunny out in Los Angeles, the perfect time for an orgasm. I grab my vibrator because if you want to start the day off right with those natural endorphins, you've got to get one in first thing in the morning! I'm a big fan of masturbation. How empowering is it that we can make ourselves cum?! Two minutes later . . . *ahhh* . . . my legs tense up and my clit is pulsing with a fantastic orgasm!

After a tall glass of water and matcha, it's 8:30 a.m., and I give my husband, Brent, a seven-second kiss before heading to the gym. Working out is vital for sexual wellness, so I make sure to prioritize it in my day. After my workout, I get ready to teach my first class of the day: Sexual Communication. I love teaching college students because they're old enough to participate in fruitful discussions about sexual well-being and very eager to learn and develop skills they'll need to live a romantically and sexually fulfilling life.

After class, I quickly glance at my phone and see a string of notifications for my newest reel, which has been shared more than forty thousand times on Instagram: "Play with her clit and watch her drip!" I smile and giggle; yes, even I get a bit jumpy hearing my videos out loud in public. But so far, it's been a great start to another day of spreading sex positivity! Then I head out to meet my fabulous publicist. As I arrive, I go straight to the bathroom and snap a quick pic of my booty and sext my husband with the message "thinking of you ;-)" At lunch, my publicist tells me that my new magazine feature about threesomes is live. Sounds great! I go home after lunch and create a reel to promote it. Before the day ends in my comfy bed, I ride my husband's face on the couch and then eat seafood pasta for dinner. What an orgasmic day!

Sounds amazing, doesn't it? But the truth is that my life hasn't always been like this. *I* haven't always been like this. There was a time when I was an anxious girl from Thailand—an immigrant trying my best to learn a new culture—uncertain about who I was or what I wanted in life. I was not sexually confident, assertive, or outspoken. I very much let cultural norms dictate my personal life. I rushed to get married in my 20s because I didn't want to be "too old" for marriage. I was extremely insecure and struggling with confidence, and I felt unfulfilled in my relationship and unhappy with my sex life. But didn't have the courage to talk about it.

Ultimately, I asked my husband for a divorce. Oh, the dreaded *D* word. I used to feel ashamed talking about it, but now I know that talking about my life experiences is my superpower. It allows me to understand and connect with people who have gone through similar trials, and I know how to come out stronger on the other side. I see divorce as an opportunity to live the life you truly desire, and now I have it: the life I love with the love of my life. It feels like a dream, but it's not. It's real.

If you've never heard of me, allow me to introduce myself. *Paper Magazine* referred to me as "the Internet's Resident Sexpert." As a passionate certified sexologist, I wear four hats. First, I'm a university professor. I'm an associate professor of sexual and relational communication (having earned tenure at the age of 33). I also teach quantitative research methods. In 2022, I coauthored the textbook *Sexual Communication: Research in Action*. As a professor, I read a lot of current research to keep my lectures up to date; grade papers; speak at conferences; and serve my students, department, and university. I've taught at the college level for more than ten years.

Second, I'm a sex-positive content creator/influencer at @Luvbites .co. I teach my fans and followers about sexual well-being, exploration, and confidence to empower them to have more fulfilling lives and relationships. With over 2.3 million followers and counting, I also help normalize frank discussions of sex and sexuality through long-form conversations with experts, celebrities, and friends on my podcast *Luvbites by Dr. Tara*. I want to help everyone feel more comfortable and confident about their sexuality and engage in open and honest sexual communication.

Third, I'm cohost of the hit UK TV show *Celebs Go Dating* (currently on my third season) and make regular "sexpert" appearances on news segments for relationship tips and trends. I love spreading sex positivity everywhere I go and whenever I can! My dream is to have my own show where I talk about sex and intimacy in an educational, funny, and refreshing way.

Finally, I have an intimacy and relationship coaching business that helps individuals and couples live more passionate and fulfilling lives. Apart from all my work hats, I'm also a loving wife, daughter, sister, and friend to many incredible souls—and, in many ways, I'm just a girl. I love getting my nails and lashes done, going out to nice dinners, and traveling around the world seeing and learning new things. One day, I want to have children, a beach house, and a Shiba Inu.

WHY I WROTE THIS BOOK

I was inspired to write this book because of my personal journey to becoming sexually powerful after my divorce. This is the book I wish I had when I was 18. I would have been so much more confident and equipped in dating, sex, and relationships if I knew then what I know now. But! It's never too late. Ultimately, if you're reading this, then I wrote this book for you. I want to help you become more sexually empowered and live the life you desire and deserve.

Sex is never just about sex. Sex is about everything else. When you embrace your sexual power, every aspect of your life flourishes, and this book will teach you how to do that. When I felt sexually disempowered, my whole life suffered; I experienced anxiety, depression, and discontent. I felt lost even though, on the outside, it seemed like I had a great life. It's true that you never really know what's going on inside someone else's head or what they're actually going through. This is why I think it's key that we not only celebrate physical and mental health but also sexual health, which is a significant part of our overall well-being as humans.

That said, the way we view sex isn't a fluke. It's a combination of who we are, how we grew up, our past and current relationships, and a lot of cultural and societal beliefs and norms. As a millennial woman of color and an immigrant who has lived in various parts of the world, I've seen firsthand how much society shapes our views on sex, love, nudity, and marriage. My diverse personal and professional experiences put me in a unique position to be able to understand and help people from all types of backgrounds.

Unconfident about your sexuality? This book can help you. Don't know how to communicate your sexual needs? This book equips you with the skills. Want to sexually explore and experiment? This book provides lots of options. Want to feel more sexually connected with your partner? This book shows you various ways to enhance your sexual connection. I think you get it—whatever your needs, this book will help you!

Although I'm more known for my out-of-pocket, thirty-second sex-ed content, I'm still a proud academic and research-based practitioner. Therefore, in this book, you can expect peer-reviewed studies, credible research, and vetted statistics that are told in an accessible, funny, and relatable way. I wrote this book with a "How can I make it not boring?" mindset, so I included plenty of real-life stories, approachable activities, ready-to-use examples, and unapologetic and hilarious personal remarks. In addition, this book introduces new trends and nontraditional perspectives on sex, dating, and relationships. One such trend in the sexual wellness space is determining your sexual characteristics.

"Help! I don't think I'm sexually compatible with my fiancé, and we're getting married in two months!" This came from a panicked client who came to me for a sex and relationship coaching session. Unfortunately, she's not alone. Millions of people experience sexual incompatibility in their relationships, which can lead to relationship dissatisfaction and breakups or divorces. Many people are familiar with their generic personality type (such as an Enneagram or a zodiac sign), but they may not be aware of their sexual profile. Wouldn't it be helpful to have a tool like a personality test but with a sexy twist so you can know more about your sexual self? Say hello to Dr. Tara's Sexual Profile Quiz (page 32), which helps you uncover your true sexual preferences and determine compatibility with your partner(s), increasing your chances of having a fulfilling relationship.

This book is divided into three main sections that represent how we engage with our sexuality as a whole:

1. **Intrapersonal factors (YOU), which include identifying your sexual profile, increasing your sexual self-esteem and sexual mindfulness, learning essential sex facts, and exploring kinks.**

2. **Interpersonal factors (YOU + THEM), which include how to talk about sex regularly; how to communicate your desires during sex in hot and nontraditional ways, using sex toys and technology to enhance your sex life; and how to understand your sexual fantasies.**

3. **Cultural/Societal factors (YOU + THE CULTURE), which include learning more about healthy and unhealthy porn consumption, how cultural and societal norms work against building passionate relationships, how not to have a sexless marriage/long-term relationship, and how to explore nontraditional relationship types without shame.**

The chapters that follow question and challenge the notions of what we as individuals have internalized, and they deconstruct societal standards about sex. Why do most people have low sexual self-esteem?

Why am I not attracted to my spouse? Why is monogamy the only option for long-term relationships? Why don't we hold ourselves accountable for a mediocre sex life?

Let me be clear: *How Do You Like It?* is meant to be inclusive of all people and all relationship types. Whether you're in a monogamous, open, polyamorous, or monogamish relationship—and whatever your sexual profile is—you'll find this book naughty, informative, and refreshing. It's time to go on this awesome journey and develop your sexpertise!

WHAT YOU'LL GET FROM THIS BOOK + SO MUCH MORE

- **A better understanding of your sexual self**
- **Higher sexual self-esteem**
- **Skills to practice sexual mindfulness**
- **Enhanced sexual confidence**
- **Knowledge of kinks and fetishes**
- **New skills to enhance sexual communication (i.e., how to talk *about* sex and *during* sex)**
- **Ideas for how to sext your partner**
- **More confidence using sex tools and toys**
- **Encouragement to use your sexual fantasies to your benefit**
- **A better understanding of how societal beliefs have affected your sexuality**
- **More satisfying and fulfilling romantic relationships**

On a sincere note: Even though I teach these topics at the university level and am writing this book based on copious amounts of research I've reviewed, alongside my personal and professional experiences, I want to be transparent that there are of course sex-related topics I don't have in-depth knowledge of—or that I mainly know from academic perspectives and not deep personal experiences. For example, I can discuss domination and power play from an informed position, but I'm not a professional or practicing dominatrix.

With that being said, consider this book like a rocket to (sexuality) space. It will be fun, informative, exciting, and new—but you won't be visiting "deep space." If you're interested in diving deeper on a particular topic, I have plenty of resources I'd recommend. Additionally, new statistics and research findings are being published regularly, so what we know to be true in this moment might be different five years from now. Nevertheless, the core of human sexuality, pleasure, and sexual connection will not change. Keep an open mind and enjoy the ride!

Chapter 1

What's Your Sexual Profile?

Who we are in bed is who we are in life.

—Samantha Jones, *Sex and the City*

Who are you sexually? Most of us don't think about who we are as sexual beings or lovers, even though sex is the most natural thing that humans do. Along with eating, sleeping, and socializing, humans have always been fucking (or love making, if that's what you like to call it). Whether that fucking is actually *good* depends on many factors. In my experience, knowing who I am sexually—and what I look for sexually, within both myself and my partners—has had a huge influence on my sexual confidence and self-esteem. I now embrace sex with fewer inhibitions, and I express myself more authentically, which has led me to having mind-blowing, leg-shaking, sex-craving orgasms—the kind of sex that 22-year-old me had always dreamed of but never had.

That's why I want to invite you to get a close and personal look at your own sexual profile. You'd be surprised how much easier it is to talk about sex with your lover, friend, sister, brother, or—dare I say—parents after reading about sexual profiles. It's a great sex conversation starter with practically anybody (although maybe not your priest). What I've seen is that it creates a butterfly effect where the person you talk to starts talking about it with others, and then *bam!* The next thing you know, you've created a more sexually awakened community. Look at you, a sex-positive influencer!

Are you consistent or dynamic? Traditional or kinky? Monogamous or flexible? Gentle or animalistic? Many people's first response when I ask them about this is "But Tara, I'm all of them!" To be sure, we *can* be all of them, but that doesn't mean it's our true and most authentic sexy self. When you think about it and dig deeper, you may find that one trait speaks to you more than another. For example, I can enjoy the same kind of sex (consistent), and I do most of the time, but I ultimately enjoy variety in my sexual encounters (dynamic). My sexual profile is dynamic, kinky, flexible, and animalistic. *Dynamic* means I crave variety in my love making. I may want loving, passionate sex one day and then want to get choked and slapped the next day. *Kinky* means I like nontraditional stuff, and we'll talk more about what that entails later in this chapter. If you're down for a threesome or sex party, then you're *flexible*, which I am. I'm not in an open relationship per se; it's more like I'm open-minded to occasional sexual exploration with others because I'm monogamish (more on this in Chapter 13). If you enjoy intensity rather than romantic and sweet sex, then you're like me: *animalistic*. Therefore, my sexual profile in a nutshell is DKFA. It's like a Myers Briggs indicator (I'm ENFJ, wbu?) but with a sexy twist. And now you know me—quite intimately.

By this point, you've probably already learned more than any high school sex-ed class ever taught you about your sexual self. Most of us are royally fucked when it comes to proper and useful sex education. Understanding your sexual profile matters because it's the foundation of everything you enjoy with respect to sex and it's never too late to learn more about yourself and become sexually powerful. I was almost 30 when I embarked on this sexual awakening journey myself, and I've been thinking about it, studying it, talking about it, and learning more about it every day since.

As a curious sexpert, I've always wondered: Is our sexuality super complex or have we just complicated it to the point where most people don't feel motivated to understand it? Why has sex become a chore? I want to change that perception, and I want you to come on this awesome and fun journey with me. Understanding your sexuality can be easy, positive, and fun. Yes, fun! Are you excited to learn more about your sexual profile? Are you a tiger, a horny rabbit, a kinky unicorn, or an empress? Let's find out!

THE FOUR DIMENSIONS OF DR. TARA'S SEXUAL PROFILE

I once had a client who told me her ex loved romantic sex. He liked kissing her for a long time and grinding on her slowly when they had penetrative sex. It was the way he loved making love. She honestly enjoyed it for a while, but after a few months of Marvin Gaye's "Let's Get It On" kind of sex, she missed getting Fucked (the capital *F* kind). She missed rough, hair-pulling, dirty-talking, animalistic sex. For her, sex became dull and, ultimately, their relationship didn't work out—not only because of the sex, but it definitely was a major contributing factor.

Millions of people around the world have had or are having the same experience. The relationship is fine, but the sex is meh. It's a universal and global experience that doesn't discriminate based on gender, culture, racial background, sexual orientation, or religion. I've talked to people from Texas to Bangkok to Dubai, and this sexual mismatch and the lack of skills to talk about it exist everywhere. Sexual incompatibility is one of the most common reasons for resentment in long-term relationships (nobody likes that), cheating, breakups, and divorces. It's time that we do something about it.

I want you to take charge of our own sex life, and the first step is to identify your sexual profile. Let me take you on a sexual awakening journey. I'll hold your hand or slap you, depending on what you like!

I'M SINGLE. WHY SHOULD I KNOW MY SEXUAL PROFILE?

If you're single and in this modern dating (mine)field, you've probably met and dated people who were not very compatible with you in terms of personality, life goals, and, of course, sex. When you're dating, sexual incompatibility is worse than other types of incompatibilities—such as not liking someone's "energy," political affiliation, or personality—because you've gone through so many hoops to get to the point of finally having sex. Most likely, you've vetted their intentions, made sure they're not a serial killer, found them attractive, and finally felt comfortable having them touch you. So at this point, your brain goes, "I'm ready for sex!" But then you have the . . . *drumroll* . . . DDA (disappointing dick appointment). A DDA means you finally have sex with someone you were attracted to, but damn, the sex was just blah. It was just mediocre sex: no sparks, you weren't in sync, your teeth smack while kissing, the list can go on, but you get the idea. And this isn't an exclusive experience for women; men have had plenty of disappointing hookups too. Actively dating in this day and age means you're bound to experience a few DDAs and disappointing hookups.

I had many DDAs in my early 20s, but not anymore. One of my life's mottos now is *No Mediocre Sex*, and it's been a game changer. I've dated so many attractive people who were not sexually compatible with me, and it sucked. Hell, I even married one, and sure enough, it didn't work out.

It can be so disheartening when you're dating someone who's perfect on paper only to find out that you're sexually incompatible. Well, I'm here to help! Before you invest a lot of energy and effort into dating someone, you deserve to know whether you have a chance for Michelin star–level sex or are bound to have fast-food sex. Ultimately, identifying and understanding your sexual profile will help you find a more sexually compatible partner! And if your date also takes this quiz, you'll find yourself treading more intelligently around potential DDA bombs.

I believe sharing one's sexual profile will become a dating norm in the future, especially when it comes to online dating. Think about it: People would be messaging each other on a dating app like . . .

Tasha: What's your sexual profile? I'm DKMG :)

James: Interesting! I'm DKMA, but I think we'll get along well ;)

. . . at least sexually, they will.

When I was single and actively dating, I always wondered what my dates were like as lovers, but I couldn't have known that without actually having sex with them. Since we don't have Yelp reviews of people, Dr. Tara's Sexual Profile is your best bet to at least establish a baseline of sexual compatibility if you're single and ready to *reaaally* mingle.

I HAVE A PARTNER. WHY SHOULD I CARE ABOUT MY SEXUAL PROFILE?

For those of you in a couple, Dr. Tara's Sexual Profile will help you better understand yourself and your partner on the sexual front, and knowing each other's sexual profile can improve your sex life. Do you know your partner sexually? Are they the type of person who would like to try pegging or rimming, or are they more likely to enjoy blow jobs and missionary sex? Honestly, don't feel bad if you don't have an answer to that question; we were never really taught to care about these things. But you're reading this book now, which means you're ready to take leaps into becoming sexually awakened, which is an incredible place to be. Yeah, you! You sexually liberated lover!

After you've learned more about yourselves, it's time to talk about what you learned. Any sexologist will tell you that communication is the key to a happy sex life. When was the last time you and your partner talked about sex? Dr. Tara's Sexual Profile can help you get started with having healthy conversations about your sexual preferences and prioritizing your sex life a little bit more, which contributes to your long-term sexual satisfaction. I guarantee that once you know each other's profiles, you'll better understand where both of you are coming from and find ways to fine-tune your sexual behaviors for a more fulfilling sex life.

Claire, who has been with her husband for five years, once told me, "OMG Dr. Tara! When we learned that I'm STMG and he's DTMA, it made so much sense! I've always wondered if I was normal because when we have sex, I only want to ride him. That's how I orgasm. It's the only position I like, but he always wants to change to different positions every time. I thought I wasn't good for him, but now I know why!"

Jake, who has been dating his girlfriend for eight years, had a similar experience. He told me, "Holly was always more intense than me during sex. I like making love to her slowly and romantically, but it felt like she was pushing me to be more 'aggressive.' Well, now I know why, and it's good to know that it's a part of her sexual profile and not that she thinks my love-making skills suck!"

These are just two examples of many testimonials from clients and friends that show how incredibly helpful it can be to understand your and your partner's sexual profiles—not only for yourself but also for your relationship satisfaction for years to come. Let's dive in!

DIMENSION 1: CONSISTENT OR DYNAMIC

Most of the time, how do you enjoy sex? Do you enjoy having variety and changing things up regularly, or do you have your go-to position and place that you always prefer?

Consistent means you have a sex ritual, and you enjoy the same kind of sex most of the time. You like comfortable, reliably orgasmic, nice sex. You're the kind of person who enjoys one or two sex positions forever and uses them to your orgasmic advantage. You tend to think, "Why change it if it's not broken?" I feel like the world shames people who enjoy consistent sex (as if it's not hot and only for boring people), but I'm here to tell you that there's nothing wrong with you. You're not boring for loving the same kind of sex for the rest of your life.

I have a yogi friend who uses a beautiful analogy to compare the Consistent sexual profile with yoga, and it makes a lot of sense. She said, "I'm a yogi. I love yoga. I can practice yoga daily and never get bored. I'm not a CrossFit kind of person. Can I do it once a while? Absolutely. But why do I need to do it when I know I love doing yoga?" That's my friend, Cynthia. She's in her mid-40s. She's been having the same kind of sex with her husband for the last fifteen years, and they love it. They usually schedule one sex night and one sex day weekly by putting it on their shared Google Calendar. She swears by it and says it brought them closer together and allows them to look forward to those times with certainty. When they have sex, she starts by giving him a blowjob, then he goes down on her until she orgasms clitorally, then they proceed to having penetrative sex in either the missionary or cowgirl position. Both of them have found pleasure in this sexual routine for the last fifteen years. They love it. Stability is how they keep their passions alive.

A Consistent Lover in Three Statements:

1. **I love consistency rather than changing it up when it comes to sex.**
2. **I love having sex the same way I know is pleasurable for me.**
3. **I love having sex in the same place I find comfortable.**

Dynamic means you love and prefer sexual variety. You like trying new things, or, when you're in a sex session, you like doing a combination of different things. You want to have sex in bed, on the couch, on the kitchen counter, in the car, on a hike, and—if you don't get caught—on an airplane to earn your mile-high-club card. Having a dynamic sex life is important to you, and the prospect of trying different things turns you on. This should not be confused with being kinky because the variety you crave can still be traditional (such as trying different sex positions within the realm of conventional sex).

If you're a dynamic lover, having the same kind of sex every single time makes you feel bored, uninspired, and nonsexual. You don't feel stimulated or aroused. You're not excited by the prospect of sex and not motivated to initiate it with your partner. Interestingly, I've found that there's a correlation between being a dynamic lover and being culinarily adventurous. Do you enjoy trying many different types of foods, or do you tend to want familiar comfort foods most of the time? I'm personally a dynamic lover. I enjoy consistent things too, but I love variety when I have sex. I might crave loving sex with my partner one day, where he says I love you, goes slow, grinds, and whispers how pretty I am in my ears; but another day, I might want him to call me a bitch, pull my hair, make me feel used, and put a butt plug in my ass while he roughly fucks me. Certain moves make me orgasm every time, like getting fingered (important note: by a person who's good at fingering), but I'm always curious to try something new, and I have a strong desire for sexual variety. It makes me horny. For me, the prospect of variety keeps the passion alive.

A Dynamic Lover in Three Statements:

1. **I love sexual variety.**
2. **I love having sex in different places.**
3. **I enjoy changing it up during sex.**

DIMENSION 2: TRADITIONAL OR KINKY

As a sexual person, how conventional are you? Are you the type of lover who will try anything and enjoys the kinkier side of sex, or are you the type of lover who likes only conventional sex? My assistant likes to say, "If the chemistry is right, is sex happening after the dinner date, or are you down to fuck in the bathroom between appetizers and the main course?"

Traditional means you like conventionality when it comes to sexual acts. It doesn't mean you're boring; there's no shame in the vanilla sex game! It's completely cool if you love conventional sex, which can be amazing and super-hot. At this point, you might be a little confused about the difference between traditional and consistent. They're fundamentally different. Traditional is about who you are as a lover, whereas consistent is how *much* you enjoy doing the same, hopefully pleasurable things, in your sex life. For example, my friend Matt is both consistent and kinky. He's turned on by feet; he likes having sex with feet and wants to do it every time he has sex.

By contrast, Diana, who loves switching it up between doggy-style and 69, is traditional and dynamic, which means she likes conventional sex but changing it up with different acts makes her feel more aroused. The interesting correlation that I've seen among traditional lovers is that they're also low in sensation-seeking behaviors. They don't have the desire to consistently seek out unique experiences that get the adrenaline pumping. In short, they enjoy conventionality in other aspects of life too. For example, Diana takes her family to Aspen every year for a ski trip, loves eating at nice restaurants that her friends have tried and recommended, and eats the exact same breakfast every day.

If your go-to sex positions are missionary, doggy-style, and (maybe) cowgirl, if you enjoy oral sex in a traditional way (no finger in the bum!), and if a hand job and potentially fingering are in your wheelhouse—but the list pretty much ends there—then you're traditional. Think of Charlotte in *Sex and the City*. She has had some freaky moments, but she's overall a traditional lover.

A Traditional Lover in Three Statements:

1. **My favorite sex position is missionary or something along that line.**
2. **I prefer conventional sexual acts rather than the kinky stuff.**
3. **I'm proudly vanilla.**

Kinky doesn't mean you're fucked up in the head, first of all (well, most of the time anyway). I'm not talking about illegal sexual kinks and fetishes here. I'd never condone something like that. I'm talking about harmless kinks and fetishes that are totally OK to explore and enjoy. There's so much shame in our society attached to people who enjoy kinky sex or certain fetishes, even though they don't hurt anybody (except for the consensual ones that turn you on). As I always say (and many other sex-positive educators have said before me), don't yuck other people's yum.

For whatever reason, there's a stereotype that kinky people are weird, socially awkward people who exist on the fringes of society. However, plenty of statistics[1] suggest that half the U.S. population has a kink. And based on my experience with clients, friends, and sex-positive communities, most kinky people I've met are interesting, attractive, and successful. I've dated an attractive PhD who has a foot fetish and wanted to cum on my feet. I've also had a sexual relationship with a CEO who loved getting his ass eaten, and it was pretty hot.

Kinky just means you enjoy sex that's outside traditional sexual norms. What's the norm? Well, it's changed throughout history and

1. Jordyn Taylor and Milan Polk, "1 in 3 US Men Are Kinkier Now than before Covid, Sex Survey Shows," *Men's Health,* February 14, 2022, www.menshealth.com/sex-women/a38912652/mens-health-kink-sex-survey/; Justin J. Lehmiller, *Tell Me What You Want: The Science of Sexual Desire and How It Can Help You Improve Your Sex Life* (Da Capo Lifelong Books, 2018); Gabrielle Kassel, "20 Common Sexual Kinks, According to Sex Educators, and Why It's Totally Normal to Have a Kink," *Business Insider,* February 24, 2023, www.businessinsider.com/guides/health/sex-relationships/list-of-kinks.

depends on your culture, generation, sexual orientation, etc. Although it's expanded in recent years, here's a list of sexual acts considered conventional in most societies:

- **Sex positions like missionary, doggy-style, cowgirl, and 69**
- **Oral sex (in a traditional sense, no extras!)**
- **Hand jobs**

So what's nontraditional sex, you ask? Here's a short list. See if you're into at least one of these:

- **Anal-related sexual activities (including double penetration and fingering)**
- **Role play and power play**
- **Voyeurism and exhibitionism (watching people have sex or being watched)**
- **BDSM**
- **Golden showers**
- **Legal fetishes (e.g., foot fetish, latex fetish)**

Many people would say that anal sex is kinky, but that's slowly changing. Indeed, couples in metropolitan cities might add anal to their "normal sex" list. Remember, though: Even though some people have a strong tendency to enjoy nontraditional sexual acts, others enjoy missionary sex for fifty years. There's nothing wrong with either, and sexual liberation means accepting healthy kinks.

A Kinky Lover in Three Statements:

1. **I enjoy nontraditional sex.**
2. **I love having kinky sexual encounters.**
3. **I love unconventional sexual acts.**

DIMENSION 3: MONOGAMOUS OR FLEXIBLE

Can sex ever involve someone outside of your relationship? Do you think that you and your partner should only have sex with each other, or do you think it's OK to involve others under the right circumstances? Does the thought of having sex with others outside of your relationship make you cringe or a little excited? There's no right or wrong answer (and absolutely no judgment) because we live in a world of possibilities and freedom of choice. This dimension allows you to understand your true self as a part of your relationship. For hundreds of years, we were led to believe that monogamy is the only way to go, but with the staggering 40 to 50 percent divorce rate[2] (many of which involved infidelity), that's not the case. At this point, I invite you to self-observe, reflect deep inside your beliefs, and critically think about which one is more like you—without the shame and judgment from society. Either can work really well, but only when it's really YOU.

Monogamous means you believe that sex is strictly between two people who are in a committed and exclusive relationship with each other. You have zero desire in trying sexual acts that involve other people outside of your relationship. Sex with someone who's not your partner sounds unappetizing to you. Consider my friend Ashley, who only eats California rolls when we go out for sushi. She absolutely loves them. She's happy and content with one type of sushi and has no interest in trying anything else; in fact, she thinks other types of sushi seem incredibly unappealing (especially toro and uni, which are my favorites). If you're anything like Ashley, you're likely hardcore monogamous, which means you require sexual and relational monogamy.

Wait, hold up. What the heck? There are different types of monogamy?! Hell yeah! In our modern society, sexual monogamy isn't the same

2. Glenn T. Stanton, "What Is the Actual Divorce Rate?" *Focus on the Family*, November 4, 2015, www.focusonthefamily.com/marriage/what-is-the-actual-divorce-rate/.

as relational monogamy. Sexual monogamy is having sex with only one partner for as long as the relationship lasts (in other words, the one-dick-for-life philosophy). By contrast, relational monogamy is being in a romantic relationship with one person for as long as the relationship lasts. It is possible to be in a relational monogamous but sexual non-monogamous relationship. It's called *monogamish* (check out Chapter 13). However, in Dr. Tara's Sexual Profile, monogamous means you want all types of monogamy: everything with one person, your boo, and there's no shame in the monogamy game. Lots of people have been happy and fulfilled with one partner for most of their lives. Indeed, monogamy has long been the norm in human society, and it still is, even though there has been a rise in non-monogamous sexual practices among the younger generations.

Tomoko came to a coaching session with one chief concern: How could she become sexually appealing to her partner?

"Why do you think he thinks you're sexually unappealing?" I asked.

"He's asked me a few times now if I wanted to try having a threesome, and the thought of it makes me want to throw up," she replied. After a few sessions, we came to an understanding that she's a demisexual, which means she's only sexually attracted to someone she has a strong emotional bond with—in this case, her partner—and any sexual acts involving other people for her are a huge turn-off. I explained that she's a monogamous lover while her partner is a flexible lover. They could still be in a happy relationship, but there needs to be compromise.

A Monogamous Lover in Three Statements:

1. **Good sex is only between me and my partner.**
2. **I love having sex with only my partner and no one else.**
3. **Sex should always be between two committed partners.**

Flexible means you're open to sexual experiences that involve people outside your relationship. It's important to stress that this doesn't mean you can date anyone and fuck everyone. I've heard some fear-based arguments, usually from people who are apprehensive about the flexible sexual profile, who say, "Oh, that just means they can fuck whoever they want. Sounds like a recipe for a disastrous relationship!" Not at all. In fact, many people are in healthy relationships and have flexibility in their sexual experiences with others. In addition, being flexible doesn't automatically mean you're a swinger or polyamorous. There's absolutely nothing wrong with either of those relationship structures, if that's your choice. Lots of people practice ENM—ethical nonmonogamy (so many fun acronyms!)—but being flexible in Dr. Tara's Sexual Profile simply means you don't believe sex *needs* to be between two people who are in a committed and exclusive relationship. So, if you're open to or have interests in threesomes, hotwifing (this is a kink where spouses agree to the wife having sex with other men), or going to a sex party, your sexual profile is flexible. In short, you're open to different sexual partner possibilities.

There's still a huge stigma for couples who practice sexual nonmonogamy, which is why it's so uncommon to see people talking about it openly, but trust me, I know many people who are practicing monogamish. For example, Erin and Sean, who have slightly different sexual profiles, do an annual sex trip together. Many times, their trips involve threesomes or playing with another couple on a pleasure cruise, but for them it's a once-a-year thing. It wasn't easy for Erin and Sean to find a happy and exciting place for both of their sexual profiles and desires. They grew up in strict religious households where openly having sex outside your marriage was extremely taboo, but they also saw their parents cheat and get bitter divorces, so they knew the shame and guilt were bullshit—but still something they had to overcome.

Flexibility can mean so many things, and you get to decide what that looks like for you and your partner. It's a design-your-life game where you hold the controllers. I'm certain that millions of people around the world are flexible in their sexual profiles, but I also recognize that it's definitely not accessible to everybody. Hailey, who's a badass attorney in a small town in the Midwest, found me on Instagram and immediately DMed me to book a session. She came to our Zoom coaching session worried but prepared, and the first thing she said was, "Is it normal that I don't want to be trapped in a monogamous relationship? All my friends are married. Hell, some of them are actually in their second marriages, but I just don't want that kind of life. I go back and forth. Like, I do want a partner, but I like sex too much to have sex with one guy forever. Does it mean I have a fear of commitment? Can you fix me?"

Let me be clear: There's nothing wrong with Hailey that needs fixing. She's far from the only person who thinks something's wrong with her for not having a deep desire for a monogamous marriage, especially since she grew up in a small town where that's the only form of relationship everyone knows and is comfortable with. How many people in the world had to go through this combination of shame and confusion just because they have a flexible sexual profile? I hope this book is a first step toward understanding and agreement that people have different preferences when it comes to how they view and practice sexual monogamy.

A Flexible Lover in Three Statements:

1. **Good sex can involve people outside my relationship.**
2. **I enjoy having sex with my partner and other people.**
3. **Sex doesn't have to be between two committed partners.**

DIMENSION 4: GENTLE OR ANIMALISTIC

What's the most attractive way for you and your partner to express yourselves and engage with each other during sex? Do you enjoy engaging in soft and romantic ways, or do you prefer to have intense and rough sexual interaction? Of course, it's possible to like both styles—and most people do—but when you dig deep and really think about the vibe you authentically prefer during sex, and what types of interactions you find sexier and hotter, you'll find your true style. I'm naturally rough, so it was easy for me to identify as animalistic, but my friend Jenny took a while to come to the conclusion that she's gentle because, even though she's occasionally down for animalistic sex, she mostly loves sweet lovemaking. Remember, just because you identify as one thing, it doesn't mean you can't also enjoy the other. It's just not your primary style.

Gentle means you enjoy and prefer having slow, sweet, romantic sex. If the sex is good, you show it through heavy breathing or quiet grunts rather than loud moaning. You don't really like rough sex; you love romantic expressions in bed. Aggression during sex and foreplay is a turn-off for you. You do a lot of soft and gentle touching and caressing because you find it extremely arousing to give and receive that kind of touch. You love slow kissing. You would usually describe your sexual encounters as loving and sensual. Basically, it's both what you like and who you are in bed, and everybody has a natural orientation toward one or the other.

I often have this conversation in my college classroom. Sexual communication is all about how you express yourself before, during, and after sex. I often have my students share whether they're gentle or animalistic lovers. One student, Lori, shared that she hates it when her boyfriend says *fuck* and that she prefers *lovemaking* because it's more civilized and loving in her opinion.

"I love it when he makes love to me slowly and whispers in my ears that I'm beautiful," said Lori. Another student, Abby, then chimed in with

"That's so cringey! To me, hot sex is supposed to be uncivilized. Use your instinct. Let go of your inhibition and fuck my brains out. Tell me I'm a dirty slut. Let me scratch your back and bite your shoulder."

Lori laughed, "Well damn, I guess we won't be having sex then!" Just a lighthearted discussion in class on a Monday, but Lori's right. It's challenging for gentle and animalistic lovers to enjoy sex together, but there's nothing a healthy compromise can't achieve.

Consider George and Samantha. They've been together for nine years and recently got married. From our sessions, they learned that she's gentle and he's animalistic. "Wow! OK. Now I feel like we have something to work from," Samantha said with a sigh of relief. Once they became more aware about their respective styles, they felt like they could compromise better. A month later, I saw them again to gauge how they were doing. "We have gentle sex twice a week and a freak night once a week" George said while grinning.

Ah, the sweet taste of healthy compromise. Who knew relationships are so much easier when you have self-knowledge and communicate?!

A Gentle Lover in Three Statements:

1. **I love slow, sweet sex.**
2. **I enjoy romantic sex.**
3. **Good sex is lovemaking, not fucking.**

Animalistic means you enjoy and prefer having uninhibited, carnal, passionately rough sex. If the sex is good, you show it through loud moaning and maybe scratching, intense grabbing, and biting. Have you seen cheetahs fucking? That's you! Aggression during sex and foreplay is a turn-on for you. You enjoy the sensation of grabbing hard, and you think a little bit of pain can be stimulating. Soft touches are not your thing since you don't find them that arousing. You like intensity when it comes to physical touch. Good sex for you might involve impact play, such as getting your ass slapped, getting your hair pulled, or being thrown around when changing positions. Intense and sloppy kissing is your jam (which is not the same as too much tongue!). You would describe your sexual encounters as passionate, intense, and animalistic. We can say you're a fan of fucking rather than lovemaking, and that's all good. Both sexual profiles can have fantastic sex.

But don't we all love a little bit of both? Well, yes, we do. People can enjoy both gentle and animalistic sex and express themselves in both ways depending on the context. Ultimately, though, we all have a natural orientation. I'll use me as an example. I can be gentle, but I love passionate, intense, and "dirty" sex. Of course, I enjoy gentle sex, and I can cum during a sweet and loving sexual encounter, but I have the most orgasmic and memorable sexual experiences when I get to live my animalistic sex dream. It's in my nature.

I did a quick survey on Instagram with 825 participants and found that 60 percent have an animalistic sexual profile and 40 percent have a gentle sexual profile. In response to whether they'd be able to have a fulfilling romantic relationship with someone who has the opposite sexual profile, 75 percent said *yes* and 25 percent said *no*. My friend Becky said it would be hard for her to date a guy, long-term, who's gentle because of how much she likes rough sex. By contrast, my friend Bianca said, "Nah, I love me a gentle bear. A big hairy guy that makes sweet, sweet love to me and takes care of me in bed like a princess." I replied, "Interesting wording there, Bianca, but do you also treat him sweetly in bed? Remember, your sexual profile is both what you like and who you are in bed." She immediately responded, "Oh yeah, I'm not this crazy bitch in bed; I'm super romantic."

While doing the survey, I also scoured the internet to see if I could find lively discussions on this topic. Bingo! I came across an interesting Reddit discussion on r/AskWomen: *What kind of sex do you prefer?*

Gentle or rough? The answers are epic and had me giggling nonstop in a coffee shop. They perfectly represent the continuum between gentle and animalistic. "Rough sex all the way. Slap my ass, bite my neck, and suck on my boobs. That's good sex for me, always," commented one Redditor (who sounds like we could be best friends). A male Redditor responded, "I like to treat a woman gentle, even if you ask me to slap you hard. It would make me upset because I feel like my gf/wife is my princess, and I wouldn't want to hurt her in an activity that is just mutually fun."

In the end, I think we can all agree that it's definitely possible to enjoy both, which is amazing! Nevertheless, my professional and personal observations tell me that we all have a natural orientation, which is crystal clear for some and hazy for others. Again, both gentle and animalistic lovers can have great sex. One is not better than the other.

An Animalistic Lover in Three Statements:

1. **I love intense sexual encounters.**
2. **I enjoy passionate, rough sex.**
3. **Good sex is fucking.**

FAQ: BURNING QUESTIONS ABOUT DR. TARA'S SEXUAL PROFILES

Are we doomed if we don't get the same letters?

Absolutely not! Realistically, I think it depends on how much you can compromise and whether you're motivated to find and commit to erotic solutions (you'll find out more in Chapter 12). Knowing your own and your partner's sexual profile can help you have better sex. But Dr. Tara, you're asking, what do you mean by that? Well, once you know your profiles, you can be more proactive in finding sexual satisfaction together and not living in sexual limbo—not understanding why your sex isn't amazing or why you're having conflicts about sex all the time.

Having different sexual profiles doesn't mean you can't have a happy and healthy relationship. There is a myth that sexual compatibility is black and white; you either have it or you don't. That's not true. The fact is our sexuality evolves throughout our lifetime, and it is possible for partners to move toward being more sexually compatible. It just takes effort and time. Many couples I work with can find something that they enjoy both together and separately.

Remember Erin and Sean? They found a way to satisfy both their needs by organizing an all-out sex trip once a year. It allows Erin (dynamic, kinky, flexible, and animalistic) the room for her sexual imagination to run wild and satisfy her need to explore, while she and Sean (consistent, kinky, monogamous, and animalistic) enjoy kinky sex with each other in their own home the rest of the year. How did this work? They first went to Amsterdam and enjoyed two lustful threesomes with sex professionals, one with a woman and another with a man. (Sex work is legal and regulated in the Netherlands.) Then they went on a pleasure cruise for swingers. Although they didn't identify as swingers, they found that their fellow cruisemates were awesome people and very friendly. They learned a lot about themselves during these trips. Erin told me that the

MMF threesome experience made her feel even closer and more attracted to Sean. Sean also had a fun discovery that he likes playing with another woman's feet while eating Erin out.

Another couple I worked with, James (dynamic, traditional, flexible, and gentle) and Shawna (consistent, traditional, monogamous, and gentle), found an erotic solution to their sexual profile differences. Shawna, who only orgasms by riding James's dick and really only likes having sex in their king bed, was able to compromise and learned to enjoy the 69 position in the living room a few times a month. They also started roleplaying so James can explore his flexible sexual profile. Shawna finds it fun to dress and act like someone else for the night, and James gets to make love to her alter-ego, Margo. Minor adjustments but major improvements.

What if I'm one letter but want to be more like the other? (e.g., I'm traditional at the moment but want to be kinkier.)

That's totally possible, but it will take some deep self-observation. Are you truly traditional but want to push your boundaries to become kinkier because of pressure from someone you're dating or because you've been vanilla-shamed and now think being kinky is cooler? Or is it that you've always had kinky tendencies but never had the space, time, or kind of partner to explore that side of you? In short, are your motivations external or internal?

I didn't always know I was kinky, but the light-bulb moment that got me thinking I might be kinkier than I thought was the kind of porn I found myself watching. (Porn can be your friend! Read more in Chapter 10.) I was often watching different types of "unconventional" porn. Some of it was just because I was curious, but some of it truly turned me on. How unconventional, you ask? Well, sex on a public bus, gangbang dreams with people of all genders, BDSM sex parties—you get the idea. My sexual imagination can run pretty wild.

These are mainly sexual fantasies, though, which means I don't necessarily want to try everything in real life. They're just fun and arousing to think about. Still, that was the moment where I was like, "Hmm, I think I'm way kinkier than I thought I was." Since I became sexually active in my late teens through my mid-twenties, I always had traditional sex, and like I said before, there's nothing wrong with that. When I began having kinkier sex, I fully realized that my sexual profile is, indeed, kinky. One of my exes absolutely loved receiving a rim job. Yes, ladies, that's when you eat his ass, toss his salad, lick his bootyhole, do the dookie, whatever phrase suits you best. NGL, at first, I thought it was weird, but when I started doing it, I realized it's pretty hot—and I soon wanted him to do the same for me. Yes, it's unconventional, and not everyone's going to love it, but I do.

Long story short, it's all good if you feel like you've been one profile category but want to venture into another because it feels more authentic to you. Authenticity is one of the keys to an incredible sex life.

Can my sexual profile change as I get older?

Yes, your sexual profile can absolutely change as you get older because many people (though not all) accumulate more sexual experiences to inform their true sexual profiles. Although I believe our sexual profiles can change throughout our lifetime, I still think there's some stability in them. If you're a dynamic lover at heart and try consistent sex for a long time, there will probably be a point where you get bored and unmotivated to have sex. What I mean is, if you're able to truly and authentically identify who you are sexually, it will always be a part of you—whether you realize it or not.

For example, I've always identified as monogamous because I was in a series of monogamous relationships where sex was only between my partner and me. I also grew up in a sexually conservative environment that left me thinking there wasn't really any other choice. I didn't know that my interests and curiosity in having sex with others was normal. I didn't know that I had a flexible sexual profile.

We live in a world where the only sexual norm is monogamy, and many people who have different tendencies end up never exploring the full spectrum of their sexuality—or cheating on their partner because they didn't have the courage and/or language to explain how they felt. Now that I'm older and have had enough life and sexual experiences, I know that I'm flexible. I've interviewed many sex coaches and experts who are older, and what I've noticed is that the older you get, the more you realize that the best relationship is one where you're able to compromise and collaborate. If you're extremely stubborn in your own sexual ways and your partner doesn't have the same sexual profile as you, it's an indicator that the relationship likely won't work out.

Can my sexual profile change based on who I'm dating?

The short answer is *yes*, but here's a story for the long answer. Cara came to see me when she was dating a guy named Danny. They'd been dating for two years. After the first coaching session, I learned that she was a dynamic and flexible lover. She said that she and Danny would have sex in all kinds of places, try new positions, and even participates in the orgy dome at Burning Man, a renowned sex party where flexible lovers can express their sexuality and have their desires met. I remember saying, "Wow! You guys are adventurous! What relationship or sexual goals do you want to address in the next session?"

She anxiously replied, "Umm, I don't know. Honestly, I feel like I'm just trying to make Danny happy. I mean, I'm OK about it most of the time and it's fun and all, but it gets tiring for me. I just want to be with him, and I don't really want him to fuck anybody else anymore."

I answered with, "That's OK! Let's work on that together."

After several sessions of unpacking her dating patterns and long-time people-pleasing behaviors, we discovered that she actually has a monogamous sexual profile playing dress-up as a flexible lover. She was so obsessed with Danny, so she thought to herself, "Just fake it till you make it," but in our sixth session, she began crying uncontrollably and realized that it's not who she truly is sexually. Ultimately, she and Danny broke up, and she's now dating a guy who understands her authentic sexual profile. The first thing she asked him to do after their amazing first date? She said, "I really like you, but can you take this sexual profile quiz first, so I know where we stand? It's great, trust me. My sex coach prescribed it."

DR. TARA'S SEXUAL PROFILE QUIZ

OK! Now it's time for you to find out your own sexual profile. Are you consistent or dynamic? Traditional or kinky? Monogamous or flexible? Gentle or animalistic? For the following statements, take your time to think about each statement, reflect on your past experiences and your true desires, and be as honest as possible. Respond to each on a scale of 1 to 4.

---

1 = DEFINITELY NOT ME!
2 = PROBABLY NOT ME
3 = PROBABLY ME
4 = OH YEAH, THAT'S ME!

1. I enjoy changing sex positions during a sexual encounter and trying new sex positions in general.
2. I enjoy having sex in different places, indoors and outdoors—not just in the bedroom.
3. I enjoy trying new sexual acts.
4. I enjoy the same sex positions that I find pleasurable and reliable.
5. My sex philosophy is: Why change something that's not broken?
6. I enjoy having sex in one place I find most comfortable.
7. I would describe myself as kinky.
8. I enjoy nontraditional sex.
9. Kinky sex turns me on.
10. The thought of kinky sex is a turn-off for me.
11. I'm more traditional when it comes to sex.
12. I'm proudly vanilla when it comes to sex.
13. Sex is only for two people who are in a relationship.
14. When I'm in a relationship, I only have sex with my romantic partner and no one else.
15. I would never have a threesome with my romantic partner.
16. I'm open to the idea of my partner and me having sex with other people.
17. Sex is not just for people who are in a relationship.

18. I would have a threesome with my romantic partner.
19. I find sweet lovemaking more pleasurable than rough sex.
20. I prefer slow and loving sex over animalistic passionate sex.
21. I prefer soft touches over intense grabbing during sex.
22. I find rough sex more pleasurable than sweet lovemaking.
23. I prefer animalistic passionate sex over slow and loving sex.
24. I prefer intense grabbing over soft touches during sex.

YOU'RE DONE! LET'S DO SOME QUICK MATH TO SEE YOUR RESULTS. :)

CONSISTENT OR DYNAMIC?

Add up the scores from questions 1 to 3 and 4 to 6. Which score is higher? If the score from 1 to 3 is higher, it means you're a dynamic lover. (Ooh, you love changing it up!) If the score from 4 to 6 is higher, it means you're a consistent lover. (Consistency wins baby!)

TRADITIONAL OR KINKY?

Add up the scores from questions 7 to 9 and 10 to 12. Which score is higher? If the score from 7 to 9 is higher, it means you're a kinky lover. (Oh yeah, you'll try anything!) If the score from 10 to 12 is higher, it means you're a traditional lover. (You're sticking with the tried and true!)

MONOGAMOUS OR FLEXIBLE?

Add up the scores from questions 13 to 15 and 16 to 18. Which score is higher? If the score from 13 to 15 is higher, it means you're more monogamous. (It's just you and me, boo!) If the score from 16 to 18 is higher, it means you're more flexible. (You play well with others!)

GENTLE OR ANIMALISTIC?

Add up the scores from questions 19 to 21 and 22 to 24. Which score is higher? If the score from 19 to 21 is higher, it means you're a gentle lover. (Meow, meow!) If the score from 22 to 24 is higher, it means you're an animalistic lover. (Grrr, rawrrrr!)

THE SIXTEEN TYPES OF LOVERS BASED ON DR. TARA'S SEXUAL PROFILE

CTMG	DTMG	DTFG	CTFG
“THE PRINCESS/ PRINCE”	**“THE SUGAR PIE”**	**“THE HORNY RABBIT”**	**“THE SMOOTH LOVER”**
Consistent, Traditional, Monogamous, Gentle	Dynamic, Traditional, Monogamous, Gentle	Dynamic, Traditional, Flexible, Gentle	Consistent, Traditional, Flexible, Gentle
CTMA	DTMA	DTFA	CTFA
“THE WOLF”	**“THE EMPEROR/ EMPRESS”**	**“THE EXPERIMENTER”**	**“THE HONEY BADGER”**
Consistent, Traditional, Monogamous, Animalistic	Dynamic, Traditional, Monogamous, Animalistic	Dynamic, Traditional, Flexible, Animalistic	Consistent, Traditional, Flexible, Animalistic
CKMA	DKMA	DKFA	CKFA
“THE SWAN”	**“THE FIRECRACKER”**	**“THE PARTY ANIMAL”**	**“THE TIGER“**
Consistent, Kinky, Monogamous, Animalistic	Dynamic, Kinky, Monogamous, Animalistic	Dynamic, Kinky, Flexible, Animalistic	Consistent, Kinky, Flexible, Animalistic
CKMG	DKMG	DKFG	CKFG
“THE ENIGMA”	**“THE WONDROUS”**	**“THE KINKY UNICORN”**	**“THE PUSSYCAT”**
Consistent, Kinky, Monogamous, Gentle	Dynamic, Kinky, Monogamous, Gentle	Dynamic, Kinky, Flexible, Gentle	Consistent, Kinky, Flexible, Gentle

Chapter 2

Big Sexy Energy: Sexual Confidence and Sexual Self-Esteem for Men and Women

It's not just about being sexy; it's about being confident and me being confident in my sexuality.

—Megan Thee Stallion, *The Madd Hatta Morning Show*

I used to daydream what life would be like if I could show up everywhere confidently, take up space comfortably, and engage in conversations like I'm one of the most interesting people I've ever met—not in a cocky way, of course, but in a way that just exudes "I'm a sexual being and know my worth." We've all met this kind of person: someone with a formidable force of sex positivity and certainty in themselves, who's not afraid to show who they are in the most refreshing and authentic way, and who is unfazed by whispered chatter and judgmental stares. Well, now I am that girl, and since I'm not a gatekeeper, I will share how you can become that person too. I believe that sustainable sexual confidence is accessible for everybody.

Women and men may fight different battles when it comes to traits that negatively affect our sexual self-esteem, but at the base level, we all have the same basic fears—fear that we're not desirable enough, not good enough, or not attractive enough to be loved. But we need to tell that part of our brain to shut the hell up because we *are* enough, and things can get even wetter—I mean better—when we work on it. The great thing about sexual confidence is that it's not fixed like height or dick size. It's not a case of either-you-have-it-or-you-don't. It's intentionally developed and maintained. A lot of people in their early 20s may not yet have a strong sense of self-esteem. When I was 21, I used to think that if my boyfriend didn't text me for more than five hours, then he was definitely cheating on me. Looking back, and after doing some investigative introspection, I realize that came from my own insecurities and lack of self-worth. I didn't think I was worthy of being loved and having a great relationship, so I sabotaged it with destructive communication patterns. I didn't have Big Sexy Energy yet.

To have a healthy sex life and a passionate relationship, you have to develop a strong sense of self and maintain your confidence through mindful practices. This then has wider significance and eventually plays a big part in every aspect of life. When I'm sexually confident, I am more confident at home, more confident when I teach, and a social butterfly at networking events and parties. Basically, I just walk around feeling like I'm winning at life 99 percent of the time. Of course I have off days (I'm not a robot), but in general, life is orgasmic, and it's here for the taking.

This journey is all about becoming sexually confident and acknowledging that it's a process. There's no miracle quick-fix dick pill or wet pussy pill. Big Sexy Energy must be developed and maintained. It's not like getting a butt lift and *bam!* You wake up with a big butt. It's more like doing one hundred squats a day to get a nice, sexy ass. You then need to continue to maintain that juicy booty with daily workouts (yes, men, some of you have juicy booties too). It took me a few years to feel authentically sexually confident. I used to feel very self-conscious during sex for a long time. I thought about the way I smelled, tasted, and looked—and whether my sexual partner was judging me—but now I feel like a sex queen who deserves *all* the attention and pleasure.

How many times have you seen an article like "Easy Tips to Help You Feel More Confident in Bed" and the solutions include something along the lines of "Put deodorant on before you get it on." Yes, that's helpful, but you'll soon realize (if you haven't already) that it's never *just* about shaving your pussy/dick beforehand, knowing how to ride a cock or do combination thrusts, or wearing expensive sexy lingerie. That kind of confidence is what I call *bubble confidence*. It's surface-level and fragile, and it can be taken away so easily—just as soon as someone gives you negative feedback like "Gosh, I can't go down on you, your pussy/dick smells weird."

But Dr. Tara, how do you know all this? I've been studying this topic for a long time, and honestly, it all comes down to this: knowing your worth as a sexual being. Having high sexual self-esteem contributes to the quality of the sexual experiences we enjoy and helps us express ourselves and communicate our desires. This chapter covers important questions we need to ask on the road to becoming our best sexy self. What are the signs of a truly sexually confident person? What affects my sexual self-esteem? How can I build higher sexual confidence and self-esteem? And more!

SEXUAL CONFIDENCE VERSUS SEXUAL SELF-ESTEEM (HINT: YOU NEED BOTH)

"Women think I'm super confident because I have muscles, I'm a gym bro, and I can make them laugh," Peter (pseudonym) shared. "They think I'm confident because of how I interact with them and what they see on social media, but to tell you the truth, I'm super insecure about my dick. I haven't had sex with anyone since my ex broke up with me. I still don't know why she broke up with me. I don't feel like I'm enough as a lover. I don't think I deserve a loving long-term relationship because my dick is so small. She'll want to find someone else."

Peter is like thousands of men out there who have penis insecurity, which leads to low sexual self-esteem. It's super common. He's able to express himself with some confidence because he's able to fake it well, but inside, he's crumbling and has a strong belief that he's not worthy of love or a healthy relationship. At this point, you might be a bit confused. What's sexual confidence, and how is it different from sexual self-esteem? To me, the most evident part of sexual confidence is how you express yourself. You feel confident, so you act confidently. It's the external part that other people can see and feel. When people say, "I love that you're so confident," it's based on the things they can observe, assess, evaluate, and interpret. It doesn't always mean that this person actually has high self-esteem and self-worth, although research suggests they're linked to one another.

The truth is . . . we live in a quick-fix society. "Take this pill! Boom, your dick works again!" "Get lipo! Yes, all your cellulite is gone!" "Wear this bodysuit that tucks your tummy in! Wow, you look more put together!" "Men, wear hidden heels in your sneakers! Ooh, you seem taller and more confident!" Let me first say that these are just common examples from predominant cultural narratives, and there's nothing wrong with you if you've done one or all of them. I'm not in the business of shaming others. I'm a true believer of freedom and choice. If something brings you joy and you're not hurting anybody, you can do whatever you want.

But back to my point of quick-fix solutions. We live in a world where speed, efficiency, and instant gratification are what people want. People are constantly searching for the one little thing they can do to seem more confident in the bedroom. Fuck with lights on? Dirty talk? Suck his dick with your eyes open? What if I told you it's not about one little thing you can change or add; instead, it's about slowly changing your entire belief system regarding your sexuality, developing high sexual self-esteem, adopting a positive sexual attitude, working on sexual mindfulness, and communicating your sexual desires and boundaries. I know, that's a bit more work, but it will benefit you in the long run. Trust me. I was once on the other (dull) side, but now I feel sexually confident and empowered, which has led me to live an incredibly passionate life.

Answer the following *yes/no* questions. Do you feel like you're worthy of sexual pleasure? Do you feel like you deserve an amazing sex life? Do you feel like you're attractive? Do you feel good about how your body looks naked? If your partner was to go down on you for fifteen minutes, can you enjoy it and feel good about it?

If you answered *no* to at least one of these questions you may have sexual self-esteem issues. Simply put, sexual self-esteem is how you feel about yourself sexually and your sexual self-worth. If you have a negative view of your sexual self, you have low sexual self-esteem. So many people have told me they don't feel sexy, don't like their bodies, or don't think they're "good at sex." That's a sexually disempowered position: a state of being where you don't feel good about your sexual self. And I know what that feels like. I was there. The cool thing about sexual self-esteem, though, is that you can develop higher levels through different practices. (Keep reading!) As long as you're down to improve, you will.

On the other hand, if you have a positive opinion about your sexual self, you have high sexual self-esteem. Do you think you're attractive, deserving of a wonderful sex life, and worthy of sexual pleasure? If you answered *yes*, congratulations! You have high sexual self-esteem, which is impressive since we live in a world full of sexual shame. Don't put this book down, though! You can still benefit greatly from this chapter. The concepts and practices discussed here will help you maintain that level of badassery. But before we dive into these concepts, let's measure your current level of sexual self-esteem with this short quiz.

What's Your Sexual Self-Esteem Level? Let's Find Out!

Be totally honest with yourself and respond to the following statements on a scale from 1 (not me at all) to 5 (totally me).

____ 1. I AM A GOOD SEXUAL PARTNER.
____ 2. I WOULD RATE MY SEXUAL SKILL QUITE HIGHLY.
____ 3. I FEEL CONFIDENT ABOUT MYSELF AS A SEXUAL PARTNER.
____ 4. I THINK OF MYSELF AS A GREAT SEXUAL PARTNER.
____ 5. I NEVER DOUBT MY SEXUAL COMPETENCE.

Add up your scores and write down your total: ___

If your score is 5–11, you have low sexual self-esteem.

If your score is 12–18, you have moderate sexual self-esteem.

If your score is 19–25, you have high sexual self-esteem.

People with high sexual self-esteem express themselves through sexually confident behaviors and communication. (Ooh yeah, fuck me baby!). They're unapologetic about their bodies, sexual needs, and pleasures, and they're not afraid to express it. They're also sexually mindful, which you'll learn all about in the next chapter.

Signs Of A Sexually Confident Lover

- **They exude positive sexual energy, (I know this sounds subjective, but sexual energy is that indescribable feeling you experience,)**
- **They clearly communicate their desires and boundaries.**
- **They ask questions to gain a better understanding of your sexuality.**
- **They ask for feedback during sex.**
- **They listen to sexual feedback without getting offended.**
- **They are generous lovers who care about their partner's pleasure.**
- **They're open-minded and nonjudgmental.**

- **They're comfortable with their own sexuality.**
- **They embrace their body and your body.**
- **They don't fake orgasms or make sexual encounters all about achieving an orgasm.**

What Affects My Sexual Confidence and Sexual Self-Esteem Level?

Life's easier when you treat yourself like you're one of the most attractive people you know. Sounds lofty and unrealistic? Not really. It's not about being better than other people; it's about incorporating the kind of self-love that fuels your confidence. And when I say attractive, I don't just mean physically attractive. You can have an attractive personality, attractive energy, attractive intelligence, attractive talent, attractive humor, attractive ambition, attractive attitude to life, attractive communication style, and the list goes on and on. When you truly believe that you're an attractive person (by your own definition), you know your worth. And that plays a big part in your sexual self-esteem. In short, you believe that you're desirable, worthy of a healthy relationship and great sex, and capable of having it.

I remember meeting this girl, Madeline, in a gym locker room. She was plus-size, with a big smile and beautiful eyes, and she just seemed so damn confident. She had sex appeal through the roof. In a world full of fatphobia, she didn't let it affect her confidence. I vibe checked her to see what she was like and said, "Girl, I love your energy!"

She ecstatically responded, "Thanks, babe! Hope you had a good workout. It's gonna be a great day!" Amazing! She was a high-vibe person. If you've interacted with someone who just exudes a sexual aura, sex appeal, confidence, swag, vibe—whatever word you want to use—understand that that's how people subconsciously demonstrate their sexual self-esteem and confidence in real life.

So where does it come from? It's a combination of various internal and external factors. Let's find out!

BODY IMAGE

"I look fat." It's not an exaggeration that every woman—along with a lot of men—have said these words at some point in their lives. We can be so damn mean to our bodies. However, the truth is that we can't hate our bodies and be sexually confident at the same time, so something needs to change. Studies[3] have shown that negative body image is a huge contributing factor to low self-esteem. It makes sense; we live in our bodies and we show up in our bodies, and if we don't think our bodies are good enough, then we can't truly experience self-worth.

Sexual confidence is related to your general sense of confidence, but it's not exactly the same. A sexually confident person knows that they are a competent lover, and they feel good showing their body because they love the way they look. My friend Katie's sexual confidence level is as high as the Empire State Building. She's so comfortable in her own body, even though she's in a skinnier frame with small titties and a little butt. She doesn't care, and it doesn't affect how attractive she feels. In a world where millions of people are striving for the Kim Kardashian body, Katie is a firecracker who doesn't give a shit that she's got tiny boobs.

Negative body image isn't just related to weight. It's also about height, penis size, breast size, body type, hair (or no hair), facial hair, face shape, eye shape, nose shape, feet size—the list goes on and on. There are probably even people who are insecure about and hate their toes; I've just never met them. These judgments aren't limited to just our own bodies; people can also be incredibly cruel about how they see and talk about other people's bodies. A study[4] published in 2020 suggests that

---

3. David Mellor et al, "Body Image and Self-Esteem Across Age and Gender: A Short-Term Longitudinal Study," *Sex Roles* 63, no. 9–10 (July 2010): 672–681, https://doi.org/10.1007/s11199-010-9813-3; S. Prabhu and D. D'Cunha, "Comparison of Body Image Perception and the Actual BMI and Correlation with Self-Esteem and Mental Health: A Cross-Sectional Study Among Adolescents," *International Journal of Health and Allied Sciences* 7, no. 3 (2018): 145–149, doi:10.4103/ijhas.IJHAS_65_16.

4. Rahul Taye Gam et al, "Body Shaming Among School-Going Adolescents: Prevalence and Predictors," *International Journal Of Community Medicine And*

body shaming and appearance-based shaming among adolescents is still super prevalent. Ugh, imagine being 15 and hearing your peers say you're ugly or fat or both. (It hurts me even typing this out.)

We're fed a constant stream of messages about our bodies and beauty standards from a very young age. No wonder we struggle with our body image as adults! It's unhealthy both mentally and physically to hate your body. Self-love and self-acceptance are crucial. When we love and accept ourselves, we take better care of our bodies. Positive change doesn't come from negativity and shame.

What's a positive body image? It's when you love and respect your body for its unique beauty and all the things it allows you to do. It's when you feel comfortable and happy with your body and know it's attractive. Freckles on your dick? Hot! Little hairs on your butt? Cute! A little birthmark in your vulva? Sexy! So, what can we do *today* to stop being such assholes to ourselves? Positive affirmations. They work. I do them daily. I'll talk more about them later in this chapter.

SEXUAL SHAME

Sexual shame is the belief that there's something wrong with you based on your sexuality, sexual attitudes, and behaviors—including your gender and sexual orientation. (Check out Chapter 11 for a more in-depth discussion on this.) It can involve feelings of disgust or embarrassment about your sexual identity and may be one of the reasons why you have low sexual self-esteem. Almost everyone experiences a certain level of sexual shame, mostly due to harmful patriarchal beliefs and misogynistic views of gender roles so prevalent in our society (i.e., women should be submissive and belong in the kitchen, and men should just . . . fucking man up, dude!).

Research[5] has found that people with religious and conservative backgrounds are more likely to experience sexual shame. This makes sense

---

Public Health 7, no. 4 (March 2020): 1324, https://doi.org/10.18203/2394-6040.ijcmph20201075.

5. Karen A. McClintock, *Sexual Shame: An Urgent Call to Healing* (Fortress Press, 2001).

since mainstream religious texts have strict rules on sexuality that are pretty much against basic human sexual desire. For example, many Judeo-Christian perspectives hold that it's sinful to self-pleasure or have sex prior to marriage. However, things look a bit different when viewed through a scientific lens. Sex before marriage is fine. Masturbation is fine. Anal is fine. No one is going to hell. I'm not against religion or practicing your faith. In fact, I practice my faith daily through prayers and meditation, but I choose to believe in the parts that are healthy for me. Which means I can masturbate in the morning and go to the temple to pray in the afternoon.

Another strong contributing factor to sexual shame is sexual orientation—especially when yours doesn't conform to what mainstream culture thinks is "normal" or "god given." Only 7.1 percent[6] of people in the United States identify as LGBTQIA, and many queer people start to experience sexual shame from a young age, particularly if their families do not embrace their sexuality. But sexual shame doesn't choose sides. Heterosexual people can also experience a lot of shame. Many women experience sexual shame from the Madonna/whore complex, which is the idea that women must be perceived as one of these two opposing identities. They are either wife material, a good girl with an innocent face and demeanor, or they're side-chick material, a tempting bad girl with a sexy face and sensual demeanor. The former persona is "worthy" but trapped in a cage, whereas the latter is free but worthless. It's fucked up, I know.

Sexual shame can last for years and affect your presence, choices, relationships, and almost every other aspect of life. In many cases, it develops subconsciously and is rooted in widespread negative messaging around sex and sexuality in mainstream culture. What are these negative messages, and do they only target women? Hardly. The messages are universally bad for everybody, so we should make every attempt to counteract them with healthy ones.

---

6. Jeffrey M. Jones, "LGBT Identification in U.S. Ticks up to 7.1%," *Gallup*, March 14, 2024, news.gallup.com/poll/389792/lgbt-identification-ticks-up.aspx.

Shame-based messages: A man should have an eight-inch dick or he's not a man. He shouldn't "simp" on women and should treat them like trash so they beg for him. He shouldn't show emotions because that's gay. Oh, and he shouldn't like getting pegged because that's gay too.

Healthy messages: Your dick isn't who you are. You should treat people with respect, and they shall do the same in return. You can effectively express your emotions to communicate your feelings. Being gay is what makes someone gay, not these weird beliefs. Plus, pegging is fun!

Shame-based messages: A woman should keep a low body count because no one wants used goods. She shouldn't be outspoken or assertive in life or in bed. She shouldn't have casual sex, but she also shouldn't be a prude. She should only want monogamy because only sluts want non-monogamous relationships.

Healthy messages: You can fuck whoever you want as long as it's safe, consensual, and pleasurable. You should speak up for yourself in life and in bed. You should have sex or not have sex as you wish. You can desire any kind of relationship that's compatible for you.

NEGATIVE SEXUAL AND RELATIONAL EXPERIENCES

***Trigger warning*: This section discusses sexual trauma and sexual assault.**

Sexual trauma is more common than anyone ever wants to admit. It's difficult even to write about and research it. Sexual trauma occurs when you're exposed to sexual abuse, which can be any kind of abuse: emotional, verbal, physical. If you've been in a relationship where your partner threatens to leave you, tries to control you, or manipulates you, you've been emotionally abused. If you've been called a "stupid bitch," "a fucking whore," "a tiny dick asshole," or any other names that hurt, you've been verbally abused. If you've been hit, punched, slapped, or physically hurt in any way, you've been physically abused.

Considering that some form of sexual assault[7] happens every sixty-eight seconds in the United States, millions of people are walking around with trauma in their bag. What if you've never been abused, but your ex cheated on you and left you feeling empty and hopeless? That's relational trauma. Negative sexual and relational experiences of all levels can affect you negatively if you don't try to heal from it. Research[8] has found that sexual trauma is also linked to low sexual self-esteem. Particularly, adults who reported childhood sexual trauma also reported lower levels of self-esteem. This is why I recommend working through your trauma—rather than suppressing it and hoping for the best. Please review recommended resources at the end of this book regarding how to work through trauma.

FAMILY SEX COMMUNICATION

"You're saying how my dad talked to me when I was 13 is the reason why I can't orgasm?! That's absurd!" Unfortunately, it's not that far-fetched. Emily grew up in a sex-negative family. Sex negativity is an attitude and belief that all types of sex are evil unless it's for procreation (to make babies) and between married heterosexual couples. Emily's dad used to talk about how her older sister was acting like a whore, having sex with boys in high school, and that nobody would ever want to marry her. His perspective eventually cemented in Emily's head and became her own, and for the longest time, she chose not to have sex before marriage because she didn't want her dad to be disappointed. In her 20s, after she was exposed to sex-positive articles, sexuality books, and podcasts proclaiming that her (her dad's) perspective on sex was all bullshit, she started masturbating and having sex with her boyfriend. Although sex was "pretty good" with her boyfriend, Connor, her daddy's voice was

7. "Scope of the Problem: Statistics," RAINN, www.rainn.org/statistics/scope-problem.
8. Emily L. Barnum and Kristin M. Perrone-McGovern, "Attachment, Self-Esteem, and Subjective Well-Being Among Survivors of Childhood Sexual Trauma," *Journal of Mental Health Counseling* 39, no. 1 (January 2017): 39–55, https://doi.org/10.17744/mehc.39.1.04.

still in her head and subconscious, making it hard for her to experience orgasms either by herself or with a partner.

Family sex communication, in a nutshell, is how your parents talk about sex—and how that talk creates a positive, neutral, or negative atmosphere about sex within the family. Our parents transmit their sexual beliefs, values, and expectations on us. For example, if you grew up in a home that considered sex to be dirty, taboo, and something you shouldn't do until you get married (unless you want to go to hell or get pregnant and be perceived as worthless), then you probably grew up to have a fair bit of sexual anxieties and low sexual self-esteem. Fear-based communication from your parents, when it comes to sex and sexuality, can negatively affect you for a long time. By contrast, if your parents talked about sex in a way that was informative and—dare I say—empowering? Then you're more likely to have higher sexual self-esteem and agency over your body and your sexuality. Studies[9] confirm this link.

At this point, you may be thinking "Shit, I'm helpless." No, not at all. Like I said before, sexual self-esteem can be developed at any age and at any time. You can always choose to embark on your sexual empowerment journey in your own time.

SEX KNOWLEDGE AND SKILLS

In my teenage years, I had "sex" with boys and girls who were clueless (myself included). It wasn't amazing sex; it was just . . . sex for the sake of thrills and novelty. When you're a teenager, you're horny. Your hormones are wild, and your body is developing. Facial hair, bigger balls, thicker pubes, the list goes on. Young people are curious animals, and they just want to explore, but you don't know what you don't know. That's why most people report that their first time having sex isn't great or memorable. Like everything, sexual competence comes with knowledge and experience.

---

9. Dalmacio Flores and Julie Barroso, "21st Century Parent-Child Sex Communication in the United States: A Process Review," *Journal of Sex Research* 54, no. 4–5 (January 2017): 532–548, https://doi.org/10.1080/00224499.2016.1267693.

That doesn't mean you have to have sex with more than a hundred people to become "good at sex." You can acquire the skills in so many different ways: reading, listening, and watching sex-positive content as well as talking about it with your friends and partner(s). Having sex is also great practice.

Experience mostly comes with age, so that is usually a primary factor that influences your sexual confidence, but it varies. For many people, true sexual confidence and sexual self-esteem come after the age of 30. When I was 21, I knew I was pretty, but other than that, I didn't know shit about good sex—and I wasn't truly confident at all. That's the thing about confidence: You have to be aware, and then you have to work on it. I've had lots of sexual experiences since then—some good, some bad—but, importantly, I've learned so much about myself and my sexual preferences. I've also made an effort to educate myself about sex. Yes, part of that is for my job, but I truly enjoy it for myself. Whether it's sharing preferences about kinks or upping my dirty talk game, I love learning and having conversations about sex with my partner.

Most of us have never had *comprehensive sex education*. In fact, some of us have never had any kind of sex education at all. Fewer than half of U.S. high schools and less than one-fifth of U.S. middle schools teach comprehensive sex ed.[10] I'm a product of that statistic. I learned about sex from the three *P*s: porn, peers, and personal experience. And something tells me that you did too. It's OK; it's never too late to learn and grow as a sexual being. Adult sex ed, here we cum!

How Can I Improve My Sexual Confidence and Sexual Self-Esteem?

I'm glad you asked! That's my favorite question. I've been on a very intentional sexual empowerment journey for a long time, and I'm so excited to

10. "State of Sex Education in USA: Health Education in Schools," Planned Parenthood, www.plannedparenthood.org/learn/for-educators/whats-state-sex-education-us. Accessed 28 July 2024.

share all the research-backed exercises that I do and that can shift your perspective on sexuality in general—your own sexual identity, attitudes, and preferences—and from there, you can grow a stronger sense of sexual self-esteem and confidence.

POSITIVE SEXUAL AFFIRMATIONS (SOLO AND PARTNERED)

"Tara, that's so woo-woo. I can't do it." This is a common response when I introduce the concept of positive sexual affirmations. Isn't it interesting, though? Billions of people believe in religion and astrology (me included) or in taking certain types of supplements even without scientific proof, but oh no, not affirmations. That's too out there. Ironically, that's also how I used to think—until I learned that my brain is like a supercomputer and when I tell her the same thing every day, she will process and make sense of it as it becomes my own reality.

What do Michael Jordan, Serena Williams, and Tiger Woods all have in common? They all believe and engage in positive self-talk/affirmations. Positive self-talk is a concept often studied in the context of sports psychology and performance[11], but you don't need to be a world-class athlete to benefit from it. It's literally one of the best daily practices for all humans, and it's completely *free*. All you need is yourself and your mind to be open to the possibility that you can be what you believe in.

Research[12] has found that positive affirmations can increase self-esteem, and positive sexual affirmation is just positive self-talk in the context of sex and sexuality. I've included here some examples from my personal affirmations bank, but you can also create your own list based on all the things you want to believe in and make it more personal to you. I do these affirmations daily. They work for me, and I believe they will

11. David Tod et al., "Effects of Self-Talk: A Systematic Review," *Journal of Sport and Exercise Psychology* 33, no. 5 (October 2011): 666–687, https://doi.org/10.1123/jsep.33.5.666.
12. Fae Diana Ford, "Exploring the Impact of Negative and Positive Self-Talk in Relation to Loneliness and Self-Esteem in Secondary School-Aged Adolescents" (PhD diss., University of Bolton, 2015), 1–24.

work for you too, but remember: You have to repeat them regularly. Say or write them with conviction. Believing you can is the first step toward developing sexual self-esteem.

There are three ways to go about this. You can say one or more (or all) of the phrases out loud to yourself as you look at yourself in the mirror. You can try doing affirmations coupled with a meditation practice where you sit still, focus on your breath, and say the phrases. Or you can write one or more of the phrases every day. Journaling is a great method to engage in positive sexual affirmations.

§ I am a great lover.
§ I am a generous lover.
§ I am radiating positive sexual energy.
§ My body is sensual.
§ My mind is open to experiencing sexual pleasure.
§ My presence exudes sexual confidence.
§ My communication is clear and attractive.
§ My voice is tantalizing.
§ I am highly desirable.
§ I am highly delectable.

Partnered positive sexual affirmations can also be extremely powerful in increasing our sexual self-esteem over time. Marco, who has dealt with body dysmorphia his entire life, has only dated men who didn't give him any positive reinforcements during sex. Recently, he started dating a guy who often says things like "Your body is so fucking sexy." He told me in one session, "Tara, you have no idea how amazing that made me feel." Marco's experience is quite common. Many of my followers have told me they love giving and receiving compliments during sex, especially when it comes to a hot comment about our sexy bodies. So don't forget to tell your partner how sexy they look and how desirable they are, and hopefully they do the same for you. If not, you should have a conversation about it (tell them about this book!) because they might not know that you love receiving compliments regularly. Honest communication and feedback allow couples to have a more fulfilling sex life.

NO FILTER BODY LOVE

The thing about body love is that people think you have to get to a certain weight or body goal to love your body. Like Mary said, "I'll be happier when I'm at 150 pounds" and "I love it when I'm a size 4 or 6." It's good to have a general health goal. I support you! But body love doesn't have to wait. It can happen at any time and any size. If you're overweight and want to lose weight to become healthier, you can still work on loving your body now and losing weight simultaneously. It's also OK if you don't want to lose weight and want to grow more love for your body as is. It's not an either/or situation. You can do both. Sex is a much better experience when you love your body. When I get fucked from behind, I don't want to worry if my partner can see my cellulite or if my ass is round enough. I want to focus on feelings, sensations, pleasure, and connecting with my partner. Who cares about my cellulite when my legs are shaking from multiple orgasms?!

There are many body love practices out there. You can verbalize your feelings about your body, talk to a therapist or body positive coach, write a love letter to your body, or focus on what your body can do for you and sit with a feeling of gratefulness for it. Most important, you should never compare your body to others'. If you want to read more about body love, one of the best books about body acceptance is *The Body Is Not an Apology: The Power of Radical Self-Love* by Sonya Renee Taylor.

Here's one of the exercises I enjoy and that helps me love and embrace my body, especially in the context of sex. Take a naked picture of yourself! It can be very empowering. A picture not only captures the subject but also encapsulates the vibe and the moment. When someone is assertive and playful, you can see it in a picture. When someone is timid and uncertain about themselves, you can see that too. So let's explore that. A sexy picture can be anything from your face, one of your body parts, or your whole body. Taking a naked picture of yourself (or in your underwear) requires a lot of self-acceptance and self-appreciation, which is why I believe it's such a good exercise. Some people have never taken a naked picture of themselves before, so I know it can be challenging.

Find a private space and time, and take a picture of yourself naked. You can stand in front of a mirror and take a picture or use your phone's front camera and take a selfie—whatever you're comfortable with. Bonus points if you're open to taking a picture that's not necessarily appealing. Can you take a picture of the body parts you're insecure about and appreciate it? At the end of the day, to feel sexually comfortable and confident, you have to accept and love your body. It does so much for you.

Things you should do to your sexual body and to boost sexual self-confidence:

§ Work out and maintain regular exercise.
§ Eat a healthy diet.
§ Pay attention to hygiene, groom yourself, and keep your body clean.
§ Give your body some love with positive self-talk.
§ Feel grateful for your body.

Things you shouldn't do to your sexual body:

§ Feel ashamed or guilty of certain body parts.
§ Compare your body to a celebrity's or to someone on social media (most of them are 'perfectly' photoshopped).
§ Engage in extreme grooming to the point where it hurts your body.

ADDRESSING SHAME

It took me a long time to get rid of the shame I felt about myself as a sexual being (and it still comes up briefly from time to time). I used to feel incredibly ashamed of so many things—from a desire to experience group sex to the scent of my vagina. I'm sure many of you can relate. Now, though, I'm not ashamed at all of who I am and what I want, even when it's against the "norm." Shedding that shame has really helped me feel more sexually liberated and confident, and it has greatly improved sexual communication with my partner.

In the following exercise, I want you to write down your personal qualities, attitudes, beliefs, values, or behaviors that are "against the norm" in an effort to work toward accepting them. I'll be honest—this won't work immediately. It's not like switching on the lights, but it can be very effective over the long term (i.e., more than thirty days).

Write a "norm statement" and a "me statement." In the former, write one of your personal characteristics, attitudes, values, beliefs, or behaviors that you experience shame around. In the latter, try to accept yourself and your own desires. For example, here's what one of my clients came up with:

Norm statement: People my age are in monogamous marriage.

Me statement: It's OK that I desire a flexible relationship, and I'm deserving of a relationship I desire.

Here's another example, from a client who was ashamed of his penis:

Norm statement: You're not a man unless you have an 8-inch dick.

Me statement: I love my 5-inch penis. It's amazing and works perfectly. My sense of masculinity is not attached to my penis.

Again, addressing and overcoming shame takes time, and this is one of many practices you can do as self-care and part of your healing process. The next step is to live more aligned to your newly accepted beliefs and values. How to do this? The first client started being more honest about what she wants on dating apps by indicating her relationship orientation as polyamory in her dating profile. The second client stopped trying to find medications and remedies to increase his penis size.

You've got to say it to believe it—but you've also got to start putting your new values into action.

REFLECT AND REFRAME NEGATIVE PAST EXPERIENCES

Important: If you've had an extremely traumatic experience, it's best that you heal with direct help from a professional, whether that's a therapist, coach, or group healing session. The following exercise is suitable for people who self-identify as someone who has had negative relational and sexual experiences but not extreme trauma or PTSD.

Have you ever been unexpectedly dumped or cheated on? Have you ever felt used? Have you ever tried to compromise and communicate with your partner but were treated with silence? Unfortunately, negative experiences can stay with us for a long time and continue to influence our sexual behaviors. In fact, after working with my therapist in my late twenties, I learned that the way I approached relationships (at the time) was pretty much influenced by my first heartbreak. I honestly didn't know that a heartbreak when I was nineteen could be that impactful in my adult life. Since that heartbreak, it was really hard for me to focus on dating one person because I "didn't want to put all my eggs in one basket." I lost my ability to trust people who wanted to date and have sex with me, so I mindlessly dated and had sex with a lot of people.

That heartbreak—and other experiences afterward—affected my sexual self-esteem for a long time. I felt like because my ex didn't want me, I wasn't worthy of true love or even a healthy sexual relationship. I had to reflect back and reframe my negative past experience in order to move on with a positive mindset about my sexuality. If you've had similar experiences, this is a great exercise to help you reframe your past and empower your future.

For this exercise, take deep breaths and reflect on one sexual or relationship moment in the past that you feel has affected your sexual self-esteem. Take your time. Don't rush. It might take a while for it to come through, especially if the event happened a long time ago. Write it down. Recalling and confronting your memory means you can benefit from a true understanding of your sexual self. Once you have that down, think of two or three lessons you were able to learn from that situation. Thank yourself for learning and growing. You can say "I'm proud of myself for having a growth mindset. I love learning and growing." (Review more aftercare strategies at the end of this chapter.)

ACKNOWLEDGE YOUR PARENTS' LIMITATIONS AND MOVE ON

I grew up in a loving household. My parents are amazing, and my mom is still one of my idols. At the same time, my parents never talked to me about healthy sex or relationships during my developmental years. Therefore, when I started sexually exploring during my teenage years, I didn't really have anyone to talk to about my sexual urges, interests, thoughts, and experiences. When it came to sex and relationships, teen Tara felt alone and insecure most of the time. I can either be mad at that today, as a 35-year-old woman, or I can acknowledge that they did the best they could and move on. I chose to acknowledge my parents' limitations and move on. I don't need to hold on to resentment or anger toward them, especially when those feelings don't serve me in any way. When you become a parent (if you choose to), you can break the cycle and start having healthy and open-minded conversations about sex and relationships with your own kids. You can also be an agent of sex positivity with your siblings, cousins, nieces, and nephews. It only takes one person to change the "no healthy sex conversation" cycle. Positive family sex communication can help young people build stronger sexual self-esteem and sexual agency in making the right choices for themselves.

I practice forgiveness meditation to acknowledge my parents' limitations and move on. This isn't terribly effective if you only do it once. You need to commit yourself to it, but after a while, you will start to feel more compassion and understanding for your parents (which in turn will build your own agency and confidence). Start by finding a comfortable spot to sit down and close your eyes. Take deep breaths and continue to do so throughout this session. Reflect on what your parents weren't able to do for you and what you wish they would have done. Then say, "I forgive you" out loud. Shedding any resentment you may have for your parents is a huge step toward developing strong sexual self-esteem.

SEX EDUCATION PRACTICE

Practice makes perfect? Not always. I've had sex with people who have had "a lot" of sex, and they weren't good lovers—even though they had a lot of practice. If they never worked on their sexual self-esteem and sexual mindfulness, they could have had sex a million times and still just be mediocre. I don't believe in perfection, but there's no denying that education and mindful practices positively influence your sexual confidence and self-esteem.

So what does sex education look like when you're not in school? Today, there's plenty of sex-positive content and sex education on the internet, and most of it is free—just google it. As always, you will need to evaluate if the sources are credible and the content was mindfully created. If the title is anything like "How to be a good woman and please your man so he doesn't leave you" or "How you can be an alpha male in bed by not going down on her," that's trash sex education. Toss it and don't look back.

Here are a few criteria to figure out if a resource is good or trash. Is it written or produced by credible creators? Research their experiences and credentials. Does it include diverse stories and perspectives? Is it intentionally dividing people in a clickbait-y way? For example, a podcast episode on "Here's why women suck" can be heavily divisive and, to me, not worth listening to. Is it obvious propaganda? For instance, if you come across a shame-based resource titled "You should never have sex before marriage," recognize its biased perspective and that it's potentially propaganda you should stay away from.

One of my favorite ways of consuming sex-positive content is by listening to podcasts. That's why I'm so passionate about producing

Luvbites by Dr. Tara, which recently surpassed three hundred episodes! My other podcast recommendations are *Sexology*, *Sluts & Scholars*, *Sex and Psychology*, *Girl Boner Radio*, *Shameless Sex*, *Sex With Emily*, and *The Bad Girls Bible*. This is just a short list. I'm sure there are more awesome podcasts on sexuality out there. You can read sex-positive books and articles. If you google "How to have a better sex life," you'll get *billions* of results, so you have tons of options (but it's essential to evaluate the sources). There are also amazing sex books from credible authors that I think every human being should read: *Come As You Are*, *Becoming Cliterate*, *Sex Talks*, *Mating in Captivity*, *The Ethical Slut*, *Sex at Dawn*, *She Comes First*, and *Butt Seriously*. Again, there are many more qualified books out there; this is just a short list. Not a fan of reading? Audiobooks are also great. You can become more sexually competent while driving, cleaning, running errands, exercising, or doing chores. Like, "OMG! I learned all about anal orgasms while I ran a mile on the treadmill, what a winning Monday!"

When you have more information and knowledge, you'll start to feel more sexually confident. Self-knowledge (knowing more about yourself) is also important when you're trying to build a strong sense of sexual self-esteem. Here's a good practice: Write down your likes and dislikes when it comes to sex. Start with your preferences when it comes to types of touch and areas of the body. For example, I like ass massages and heavy grabbing. I don't like hard spanks on my ass. I like kissing with a little tongue; I don't like sloppy kisses. I like getting my ass eaten, but I don't like a finger in the butt without a proper warm-up. I like smooches on the neck, but I don't like someone licking my neck. You get the idea. Now it's your turn! Only you can put yourself in a sexually empowering position to have that Big Sexy Energy!

Important Note on Aftercare

Many of the exercises in this chapter can feel hard and heavy. After completing each exercise, it's important to check in with yourself to see how you're feeling and try some aftercare practices. For instance, focus on soothing visuals to end a session. This can be a loving picture of yourself with your friends or family or a fun selfie where you exude happiness and confidence. You can also end a session with comforting scents, such as a candle you love or other essential oils. My favorite is eucalyptus, which I find very calming and smells like home. Keeping a diary of your self-reflections after these exercises can also be helpful in understanding your journey and how far you've come. Always remember, your sexual powers are in your hands and you're capable of creating positive change within yourself.

Chapter 3

Fucking Mindfully: Upgrade Your Sex Life with Mindfulness and Tantra

The more whole we are as sexual beings, the more fulfilled we are as human beings.

—Amy Jo Goddard

The best fucks of my life are when I'm in the moment, am not distracted by anything, and can feel *everything*. My clit is throbbing because my partner just licked it until I came. My vagina is pulsating because he's fucking me with conviction, and I can feel his hard cock stroking in and out of my pussy in perfect tempo. My neck is tingling because he's kissing it. My palms are sweaty from all this horniness. I'm able to feel all of this because I practice sexual mindfulness. But what the hell is sexual mindfulness? It's the state of being completely conscious and present during sex without the feeling of judgment for yourself or others. It's being 100 percent immersed in the moment. When you're sexually mindful, you can feel everything more intensely, which means a more fulfilling way to experience pleasure.

Sexual mindfulness is definitely not a new concept. Over the years, it's been taught and called different things, such as tantra or tantric practices. It can be dated back thousands of years and wasn't originally associated with sex. The purpose of practicing nonsexual tantra was to gain a deeper sense of self-awareness and connect with your spirituality. The origins of tantra[13] are in an ancient Indian philosophy and practice that encompasses various interpretations of principles and mindfulness practices such as breathwork, yoga, and meditation.

In 2010, researcher Vikas Dhikav and colleagues [14] conducted an experiment by enrolling women in a yoga camp and then asking them about their sexual functioning afterward. They found that after doing yoga for twelve weeks, participants' sexual functioning significantly improved. This included enhanced desire, arousal, lubrication, orgasms, and satisfaction. In the same year, Dhikav and colleagues [15] also studied the effects of yoga on men's sexual functioning. They found that yoga also improved men's sexual function, including desire, satisfaction, performance, erections, orgasms, and ejaculatory control. Amazing, right? It's safe to say that yogis are some of the best lovers because they practice being present through breath and body while also enhancing their mobility and agility.

The tantric practices I'm talking about in this chapter are great for your mental, physical, and sexual health. That's probably why there have been an increasing number of tantric sex teachers and entrepreneurs over the years. There has been criticism that tantra objectifies women, but I love Dr. Loriliai Biernacki's interpretation in *Renowned Goddess of Desire: Women, Sex, and Speech in Tantra* where she states that women are actually revered and worshipped in tantra, a powerful and connecting concept for people of all sexual orientations.

Although the concept of sexual mindfulness is mostly a Western one, the main aspects of it are rooted in tantric principles and beliefs. Sexual

---

13. David Gordon White, *Kiss of the Yogini: "Tantric Sex" in Its South Asian Contexts* (University of Chicago Press, 2006).
14. Vikas Dhikav et al., "Yoga in Female Sexual Functions," *Journal of Sexual Medicine* 7, no. 2 (February 2010): 964–970, https://doi.org/10.1111/j.1743-6109.2009.01580.x.
15. Vikas Dhikav et al., "Yoga in Male Sexual Functioning: A Noncomparative Pilot Study," *Journal of Sexual Medicine* 7, no. 10 (October 2010): 3460–3466, https://doi.org/10.1111/j.1743-6109.2010.01930.x.

mindfulness is not yet mainstream, but I want everyone to know about it. Sharing is caring, and happy girls don't gatekeep. I believe we can all benefit from it, so here I am, dedicating a whole chapter to this—changing the world, one leg-shaking, amazing fuck at a time.

In this chapter, I'll share my sexual mindfulness journey and what my study (which I presented at TEDx) of five thousand participants tells us about amazing sex. I'll also talk about the studies that piqued my interest in this concept, the practices that I tried—along with what did and did not work—and some clients' stories. I'll also share what I found most surprising when it comes to sexual mindfulness and tantric sex. But first, let's start with a story that I believe we can all relate to about why sexual mindfulness is the golden key to a long-term happy sex life.

One Wednesday evening, Jane came home from a day of dealing with chaos at work and handling drama from coworkers. She took her heels off and sunk into the couch. Her shoulders were tight, her neck was in pain, and all she wanted to do was fucking eat a bowl of pasta, down a glass of red wine, and go to bed. How could she be "in the mood" to have sex? Her boyfriend, Kevin, who's a professional photographer, had an amazing day shooting in Central Park and received a bunch of email accolades for his new photography feature in a local magazine. He was feeling confident, dominant, and, of course, horny. He came into the living room and sat next to Jane and asked how her day was. Jane started venting about her overly dramatic coworker and a few stressful things that were happening at the office. After she asked him about his day, Kevin started giving her a little shoulder rub while telling her about his amazing day. He started caressing her and then told her she looked absolutely beautiful and that he wanted to fuck her and give her multiple orgasms.

What do you think? Can Jane and Kevin have an enjoyable sexy session? Is it selfish for Kevin to initiate sex? Is it bad if Jane rejects him? What can they do to reconcile the desire discrepancy? Millions of people have this kind of experience every day, and there are many questions and perspectives to consider in this kind of situation. If I'm Kevin, I would ask Jane how I could help her relax and relieve stress. If I'm Jane, I would ask myself, "Aren't you always going to be somewhat stressed coming back from work? Does it serve you to continue the stress at home and consistently deny an opportunity for sexual connection that can turn into wonderful pleasure? Is it possible that you can get into a sexy mental space?" Like one of my favorite psychotherapists, Esther Perel, once said, "Sex isn't just something we do, it's a space we go . . ."[16] This is where sexual mindfulness practices can help. After a ten-minute guided sexual meditation, Jane could become more susceptible to sexual stimuli and open to sexually connecting with Kevin.

Mindfulness is defined as the state of being conscious and aware of something. You might say, "Well, I'm having sex. My body is here and I'm participating, so yeah, I'm conscious." Not always. Sometimes we have mindless sex with a casual partner or even with a long-term partner. A mindful act takes more effort and intention, which is why good sex can feel *reaaally* good. Sexual mindfulness is a term more commonly used in academia and the social scientific realm, whereas tantra is associated with the concepts of energy and the metaphysical. Whether you're making love, fucking, or exchanging energies—whether it's ten minutes, an hour, or seven hours (fun fact: Sting once told a reporter that he enjoys seven-hour tantric sex sessions with his wife[17])—the most satisfying way to go about it is to be mindful. Tantric sex encourages lovers to be present in the moment, which is why I believe sexual mindfulness and tantric sex are intertwined. Tantric sex *is* mindful sex. Both tantric sex and sexual mindfulness are applicable to solo sex (masturbation) and partnered sex. So you can use any term that is more aligned with your beliefs. They're all good—and good for you!

---

16. Esther Perel and Mary Alice Miller, "Letters from Esther #37: Eroticism Is an Art. But It's Also a Practice," Esther Perel, https://www.estherperel.com/blog/letters-from-esther-37-eroticism-is-an-art-but-its-also-a-practice.

17. ABC News, "Sting Talks 7-Hour Tantic Sex with Trudie Styler," October 23, 2014, https://abcnews.go.com/Entertainment/sting-talks-hour-tantic-sex-trudie-styler/story?id=26398064.

SEXUAL MINDFULNESS QUIZ

Sexual mindfulness is about tuning into your mind-body-breath connection. It's about being in tune with your own and your partner's body and energy. People who are sexually mindful are fully aware of their own mind-body-breath connection (e.g., arousal creation translating from the mind to the body). They're able to engage in sexual encounters and remain entirely present and nonjudgmental the whole time.

There are different levels of sexual mindfulness. Here's a little quiz to learn about your current level of sexual mindfulness. Please be completely honest with your answers. You can only benefit from knowing where you're at now and working to improve your ability to be more mindful.

Respond to the following statements from 1 (not me at all) to 5 (totally me).

____ 1. I CAN EASILY IDENTIFY WHEN I'M SEXUALLY AROUSED.

____ 2. I USUALLY FEEL COMPLETELY PRESENT DURING SEXUAL INTERCOURSE.

____ 3. I DON'T JUDGE MYSELF WHEN I OR MY PARTNER DON'T REACH ORGASM.

____ 4. I CAN EASILY HELP MY PARTNER UNDERSTAND WHAT MAKES ME FEEL GOOD OR WHAT MY SEXUAL NEEDS ARE.

____ 5. I AM VERY ATTENTIVE TO MY PARTNER AND MYSELF DURING SEX.

Add your scores and write down your total: ____

If your total score is 5–11, you have low sexual mindfulness.

If your total score is 12–18, you have moderate sexual mindfulness.

If your total score is 19–25, you have high sexual mindfulness.

WHY SHOULD I CARE ABOUT SEXUAL MINDFULNESS?

Why should you care? Because it's the golden key to a sustainable amazing sex life. *Sustainable* is the key word here. Sure, you can have a good fuck with an exciting one-night stand that's hot and spicy, but that kind of rush isn't sustainable. It goes away—sometimes faster than you'd like. I know, I've tried.

I asked myself this question when I first embarked on my sexual empowerment journey. When I first stumbled upon this concept, I thought to myself, "What woo-woo shit is this? Just throw me around and fuck my brains out." *That's good sex.* I can't deny that it still sounds like a lot of fun, but it's missing one key element: me *feeling* everything and *being* in the moment. Being more mindful means you can stay present and focused during sex longer, which is a challenge for many people.

We have up to fifty thousand thoughts a day. Can you imagine? Some are thoughts we don't want to have but still pop up in our heads. Have you ever had random thoughts during sex? That's when your mind goes elsewhere and you start to think about other things—aside from the sex that you're having. It's super common. It might be about something mundane like a to-do list (When will I get it all done?) or something spicier, like another lover.

A survey based on two thousand adults[18] found that 49 percent of people fantasize about other people during sex. I'm not surprised; I've done it many times. In the past, there were times I thought about other people fucking me during sex with my ex-boyfriend, thought about eating pussy instead of sucking dick, or thought about a sexy masc lesbian massaging my tits instead of the person I was having sex with. I've even thought about what I wanted to have for dinner and which app I should

---

18. Asia Grace, "Your Partner Is Probably Fantasizing about Someone Else during Sex: New Study," *New York Post*, September 8, 2023, nypost.com/2023/09/08/almost-half-of-americans-think-about-someone-else-during-sex-study/.

use to reserve a table. Seriously, it's way more common than you probably think, so there's no need to shame yourself for it.

However, since I started practicing sexual mindfulness, I've learned to focus during sex way more, and my orgasms have intensified and multiplied. You may have heard that an orgasm is a brain event, not a body event, meaning that your mind has to be ready and in the right mindset to experience a full-blown climax. I admit that I never had multiple orgasms until I started practicing sexual mindfulness in my 30s. It's not that an orgasm is the only goal, because it's not, but it's one of the observable benefits of sex, and I know a lot of people struggle with not being able to cum (i.e., anorgasmia).

Have you ever felt anxious as you were anticipating sex with a new partner or trying a new sexual act with your current partner? If so, you're normal. At some point in our lives, we all have sexual anxiety. Research [19] has found that low sexual self-esteem is linked to sexual anxiety, which means it has a reciprocal effect. Anxiety contributes to low sexual self-esteem and vice versa. Not everyone has debilitating sexual anxiety that prevents them from having sex. For some, it's unnoticeable, and many people experience it at a low or moderate level. Symptoms include, but are not limited to, negative thoughts and feelings during sex, an inability to orgasm, premature or delayed ejaculation, erectile dysfunction, dry vagina, painful sex, and a decreased interest in sex. There are also two types of sexual anxiety: trait anxiety and state anxiety. If you're an anxious person in every context of life, that's called trait anxiety, and it affects you in the bedroom too. If you're not anxious outside the bedroom but still experience anxiety during sex, that's called state anxiety, and it's a bit easier to deal with.

Certain situations can also cause more anxiety. For men, it's the anticipation of an erectile dysfunction or cumming too fast. For women,

---

19. Audrey Brassard et al., "Attachment Insecurities and Women's Sexual Function and Satisfaction: The Mediating Roles of Sexual Self-Esteem, Sexual Anxiety, and Sexual Assertiveness," *Journal of Sex Research* 52, no. 1 (December 2013): 110–119, https://doi.org/10.1080/00224499.2013.838744.

it's our own body image. What sexual situations cause you anxiety? It helps to pinpoint certain situations so you know where the fear comes from and then you can work toward adjusting your belief system around that fear. How can we feel less anxious before, during, and after sex? In a very practical manner, sexual mindfulness helps us deal with our sexual anxiety and its associated symptoms. Breathwork is linked to reduced anxiety, and meditation fosters the ability to be present. We know mindfulness-based therapy[20] helps with fear linked to sexual activity, sexual dysfunction, arousal, and desire, and it increases sexual satisfaction. Doesn't it feel like mindfulness practices can heal us all? To be honest, I think it can!

FIVE THOUSAND PEOPLE TOOK A SURVEY ABOUT SEX: WHAT DID WE FIND?

Sexually mindful people have the best sex life because they're more confident and can communicate their sexual desires and boundaries. A prominent Harvard study[21] revealed that good relationships lead to long and happy lives. It's the main factor that contributes to longevity and life satisfaction. Good genes may help you live longer, but having solid joyful relationships is the main predictor of a great life. So what's the role of sexual well-being in a happy relationship? Does self-perceived sexual satisfaction affect the way people feel about their own romantic relationships? Fuck yeah it does. For the last seven years, I've been obsessed with understanding the predictors of a good sex life. We know from many studies[22] and, let's be honest, personal experiences that sexual satisfac-

20. Izabela Jaderek and Michal Lew-Starowicz, "A Systematic Review on Mindfulness Meditation–Based Interventions for Sexual Dysfunctions," *Journal of Sexual Medicine* 16, no. 10 (October 2019): 1581–1596, https://doi.org/10.1016/j.jsxm.2019.07.019.
21. "Harvard Second Generation Grant and Glueck Study," Harvard Study of Adult Development, www.adultdevelopmentstudy.org/grantandglueckstudy.
22. E. Sandra Byers, "Relationship Satisfaction and Sexual Satisfaction: A Longitudinal Study of Individuals in Long-Term Relationships," *Journal of Sex Research* 42, no. 2 (May 2005): 113–118, https://doi.org/10.1080/00224490509552264.

tion is a contributing factor to relationship satisfaction. Most people feel more fulfilled in a relationship when their sex life is thriving, so I set out to figure out what factors predict sexual satisfaction.

I'm a mix of Eastern and Western influences. I'm originally from Asia, and I love learning about Eastern philosophies and practices, but I also spent six years in graduate school in the United States and love conducting social scientific research. I'm a quantitative research professor who uses statistics in studying sexual attitudes and behaviors. A few years ago, I embarked on a journey to conduct a large research study with one question in mind: What intrapersonal and interpersonal factors contribute to self-perceived sexual satisfaction? More than five thousand people from all walks of life participated in the survey, which ultimately included heterosexual people and LGBTQ folks, respondents who ranged in age from 18 to 60, and people from various cultural and racial backgrounds. One requirement to participate in the study was that they had to have been in at least one committed romantic relationship that involved sexual activities between the partners. Here were the top five findings:

1. **Sexual mindfulness is the foundation of a good sex life.**
2. **Sexually mindful people reported higher levels of sexual self-esteem.**
3. **Sexual self-esteem is strongly linked to sexual confidence.**
4. **Sexually confident people engage in sexual communication more often.**
5. **Sexual communication is necessary for long-term sexual satisfaction.**

Sexual mindfulness is at the start and the heart of every journey to sexual satisfaction. Sexual satisfaction is a big part of our overall life and relationship satisfaction, so it's fair to say that being more mindful isn't just great for your sex life; it's great for your overall life happiness.

TALK NERDY TO ME: OTHER INTERESTING SEXUAL MINDFULNESS STUDIES

Working with clients is one of my favorite things to do because you get to meet so many cool people and learn about their perspectives, their life experiences, and the choices they make. Rachel is an outspoken woman in her forties who only believes in scientific facts. As a lawyer, she never spent a lot of time looking into mindfulness. The first time I introduced her to the concept of sexual mindfulness, she laughed and said, "I'm not sure if I'm into this woo-woo BS." I took her response as a challenge to find and share as many scientific findings about sexual mindfulness as possible.

After a couple days, I emailed her and said, "Here's a review on fifteen studies about mindfulness and sexual well-being!" The paper[23] I shared with her is titled "A Systematic Review on Mindfulness-Meditation Based Interventions for Sexual Dysfunctions" by clinical sexologists Izabela Jaderek and Michal Lew-Starowicz. They reviewed fifteen studies that focused on using mindfulness to help people with sexual dysfunctions, and they found that all research indicated its effectiveness. Ultimately, sexual mindfulness exercises helped participants with arousal, desire, and sexual satisfaction. Jaderek and colleagues also conducted another study[24] in 2023 enrolling women both with and without sexual dysfunctions in a four-week mindfulness program. They found that the program positively affected *all* women. Specifically, they found that sexual mindfulness practices are positively linked to arousal and desire, sexual satisfaction, a reduction of fear related to sexual activity, and an improvement in perceived arousal and genital responses.

---

23. Jaderek and Lew-Starowicz, "A Systematic Review on Mindfulness Meditation–Based Interventions for Sexual Dysfunctions," 1581–1596.
24. Izabela Jaderek, Katarzyna Obarska, and Michal Lew-Starowicz, "Assessment of the Effect of Mindfulness Monotherapy on Sexual Dysfunction Symptoms and Sex-Related Quality of Life in Women," *Sexual Medicine* 11, no. 3 (June 2023): 1–17, https://doi.org/10.1093/sexmed/qfad022.

Esteemed researcher Dr. Lori Brotto, at the University of British Columbia[25] Sexual Health Research lab, is known for her research and expertise in mindfulness-based therapy for sexual dysfunctions. She is the author of hundreds of papers and the book *Better Sex Through Mindfulness* and has been cited more than fourteen thousand times. Dr. Brotto has found mindfulness practices to be one of the secret weapons to a better sex life. She is also one of the most badass academics/researchers I've ever met. She has a cool and calm demeanor but is passionate and energetic when she talks about her sex studies. I had the pleasure to have her as a guest on my podcast, and wow! She confirmed my belief in how important it is to practice mindfulness because it has a powerful effect on your sex life. Here are some of her most mind-blowing findings.

Meditation leads to better sex. Among women who didn't experience sexual dysfunction, those who meditate had greater sexual response (the process we go through from arousal to orgasm) and higher sexual satisfaction. In 2007, her study on the application of mindfulness in sex therapy included women who had issues with getting sexually aroused. Specifically, they had sexual arousal disorder from gynecologic cancer, so it was hard for them to get aroused or enjoy sex. After participating in the intervention, they felt that mindfulness improved their sexuality and quality of life. A 2008 paper[26] highlighted the effectiveness of mindfulness-based psychoeducation. She found women participating in three ninety-minute interventions over a two-week span self-reported that their vaginal wetness improved and that they could get physically aroused more easily. She also found that among women with a history of sexual abuse, the intervention helped them improve sexual excitement and genital tingling. Aren't these findings incredible? This is why I fuck-

---

25. "Dr. Lori Brotto: UBC Sexual Health Research: Mindfulness Expert," Department of Obstetrics and Gynaecology, University of British Columbia, brottolab.med.ubc.ca/.

26. Lori A. Brotto and Rosemary Basson et al., "A Mindfulness-Based Group Psychoeducational Intervention Targeting Sexual Arousal Disorder in Women," *Journal of Sexual Medicine* 5, no. 7 (July 2008): 1646–1659, https://doi.org/10.1111/j.1743-6109.2008.00850.x.

ing love doing sexual meditation! Not sold on it yet? Let's check out more reviews of some awesome studies.

In 2012[27], Brotto again tested the effectiveness of mindfulness-based sex therapy but included a six-month follow-up. Guess what? She saw the same amazing results. The participants engaged in ninety-minute group sessions, including meditation, cognitive therapy, and education, and they showed increased sexual desire, arousal, lubrication, and overall sexual satisfaction and decreased orgasm difficulty. Another study[28] that same year also found that brief interventions, including three ninety-minute mindfulness-based cognitive behavior therapy sessions, helped endometrial or cervical cancer survivors improve their sexual functioning and reduce their sexual distress. In addition, women who experienced childhood sexual abuse participated in the mindfulness-based therapy and reported significant decreases in sexual distress.

At this point, I think you get the idea. Mindfulness is powerful when it comes to having a great sex life. A study[29] published in the *Journal of Sex & Marital Therapy* suggests more sexually mindful people (especially women) tend to have better self-esteem. The researchers studied 194 heterosexual married people 35 to 60 years old and found that sexual mindfulness has a lot to do with sexual satisfaction, self-esteem, and how satisfied you are with your relationship. Another study[30] found that mindfulness promotes sexual satisfaction and mitigates sexual insecurities in men and women.

---

27. Lori A. Brotto and Rosemary Basson, "Group Mindfulness-Based Therapy Significantly Improves Sexual Desire in Women," *Behaviour Research and Therapy* 57 (June 2014): 43–54, https://doi.org/10.1016/j.brat.2014.04.001.
28. Lori A. Brotto and Yvonne Erskine et al., "A Brief Mindfulness-Based Cognitive Behavioral Intervention Improves Sexual Functioning versus Wait-List Control in Women Treated for Gynecologic Cancer," *Gynecologic Oncology* 125, no. 2 (May 2012): 320–325, https://doi.org/10.1016/j.ygyno.2012.01.035.
29. Chelom E. Leavitt et al., "The Role of Sexual Mindfulness in Sexual Wellbeing, Relational Wellbeing, and Self-Esteem," *Journal of Sex & Marital Therapy* 45, no. 6 (March 2019): 497–509, https://doi.org/10.1080/0092623x.2019.1572680.
30. Cara R. Dunkley et al., "The Potential Role of Mindfulness in Protecting Against Sexual Insecurities," *Canadian Journal of Human Sexuality* 24, no. 2 (August 2015): 92–103, https://doi.org/10.3138/cjhs.242-a7.

Namaste, y'all! Get on with your favorite sexual mindfulness exercise. You already know it's good for your sexual functioning, self-esteem, insecurities, sexual fulfillment, and relationship satisfaction.

FIVE SIMPLE SEXUAL MINDFULNESS PRACTICES YOU CAN DO TODAY

At this point, you're probably dying to know what practices are effective and ineffective in fostering sexual mindfulness, so let's get to it. I'm sharing five easy exercises that have been proven to be effective from research, my personal and professional experiences, and other practitioners' experiences.

Sexual Meditation (Solo or Partnered)

Sexual meditation is like a regular meditation practice, but it focuses on sexual thoughts, feelings, and sensations in your body. Sexual thoughts can include (but are not limited to) memories of a previous sexual encounter, sexual fantasies you have (e.g., a cuckolding kink), or imagined sexual encounters with someone you know (or a total stranger). I have tried and loved all of them. Reliving a memory is super hot and can help you regain appreciation for your partner if you're in a long-term relationship. One memory I love reliving is a time I visited my partner in his studio on a rainy day. I wore a miniskirt and watched him paint for a little bit, but I knew he was getting horny from watching me watch him. I started opening my legs and I wasn't wearing underwear, so he could see my pussy waiting for him. I played with myself, and he immediately stopped painting. He walked over, took off his pants, and the rest . . . well, you know, it's in my memory! That's just one of many sexually stimulating memories I have. What about you? I find it easier to do this sexual meditation when I write down in my sex journal (more on this later) what moment I wanted to relive in that session.

The second type of thought is when I play out a sexual fantasy. One of my fantasies is being helplessly fingered by multiple partners. It's a complete fantasy because in real life I'm too much of a germaphobe to have that many strangers' fingers in my pussy, so I wouldn't be comfortable doing it—but in my mind? It's fucking lit! It's a total turn-on when I meditate and my mind goes to that group fingering fantasy. I have other fantasies I sometimes think about, but that's for another time. What about you? It's OK if your fantasy is taboo. What I've noticed is that lots of people experience shame related to their own sexual fantasies because our imagination can sometimes think of things you would never, ever do in real life. Remember, it's OK to have fantasies. It doesn't mean you actually want to do them IRL.

The third type of thought is imagined sexual encounters with strangers or someone you know. Imagining hot, passionate sex with a stranger or a secret crush can be super fun. Your mind can be very active if you let it run wild. One of my friends loves imagining an orgy with aliens where she gets abducted and becomes a sex slave on an alien ship. Yes, when it comes to human imagination, it can get *wild*. Just look at all the movies produced in the last fifty years. Some of them are super imaginative and weird in the best ways, so, yes, sexual imagination can also be extremely creative.

Another type of sexual meditation focuses on feelings and sensations. In other words, it's more visceral than thought-based meditation. When it comes to feelings and sensations, you can do a whole-body scan meditation or focus on a few body parts or one part per session. I like full-body scans once in a while, but for sexual meditation, I prefer to focus on a few erogenous zones. For me, that includes my nipples, thighs, and pubic area (sometimes I venture down to my pussy but not all the time because my intention isn't to masturbate). The purpose of this kind of meditation is to not only practice sexual mindfulness but also gain self-knowledge about how each part of your body feels and which parts are more arousing than others to touch and stimulate. Many people have told me this kind of meditation helps them reconnect with their bodies and allows them to experience more pleasure through touch with a partner.

Affirmation meditation is another type of sexual meditation I really like. This involves sitting still, taking deep breaths, and repeating positive sexual affirmations to yourself. You can say them out loud, quietly, or in your head. Affirmations are great at helping you increase your self-esteem, so by mixing meditation and sexual affirmations, you're learning to be more mindful and sexually confident. Every type of sexual meditation can be done by yourself or with your partner(s). It's a great daily solo practice, but doing it with your partner once in a while (or regularly) can enhance the connection and passion you have for each other. You can do it quietly or play light, sensual music in the background. If you find this too difficult to do on your own—or if you just prefer a guide in general—I have a list of free guided sexual meditations by me on YouTube that you can totally use. Sit down, press play, do what I say, and enjoy!

Mindful Masturbation (Solo or Partnered)

"OMG, I'm about to cum . . . but wait."

Everyone masturbates. I started masturbating when I was thirteen; it's pretty common to start having sexual urges when you hit puberty. It doesn't matter who you are. Regardless of where you live or your gender, race, sexual orientation, political beliefs, or language you speak, your sexual hormones and personal curiosity will inevitably express their needs. People's urges and frequencies differ quite drastically. Some people masturbate every day. Some people masturbate once a week. Some people masturbate once a month. Some people rarely masturbate.

Doctors and health educators confirm that regular masturbation is healthy for you, but that doesn't mean you have to do exactly what science says. You do you, boo! You should do whatever feels good for you as long as it's mindful and pleasurable. The art of mindful masturbation is slowly fading in today's world where people prefer efficiency over mindfulness. To that end, reliance on porn is increasing at an alarming rate. Recent research[31]uncovered the hard truth that most people need to watch porn while they masturbate, and some people literally can't get aroused without it. Does this sound like you or someone you know? If so, no worries. There's hope! A practice like mindful masturbation can revitalize your sexual imagination and the mind-body connection. You just have to be patient when you do it (I know, easier said than done) since it takes practice, but you'll get there. Mindful masturbation involves four principles: allowing yourself time, synchronizing your breath, mixing different touches, and focusing on the now.

Allowing yourself time: A vital part of mindful masturbation is that you're not rushing. Often, when we masturbate, we have one goal: cum as fast as possible because pleasure feels good. Yes, I know! I myself can cum in two minutes or less. But with this practice, you're not trying to do that; you're giving yourself permission and time to explore your body and the different sensations available to you. Whether you're stroking your cock or stimulating your clit, doing it slowly is a big part of this exercise. You can try edging, which is the practice of stimulating yourself to the point of almost cumming (bringing yourself to the edge) only to stop, breathe, and then continue. Edging doesn't always end with an orgasm, but it can! It's your choice.

Synchronizing your breath: This is all about being mindful of your breath while deepening the experience of pleasure. It's well documented that breathwork (or deep breathing) enhances arousals and orgasms because it releases nitric oxide into the body. (I'll talk more about this later when I discuss erotic breathing.) For example, you can synchronize your breathing with your hand or a toy movement, or you can sync your

---

31. N. Prause, "Porn Is for Masturbation," *Archives of Sexual Behavior* 48, no. 8 (2019): 2271–2277, https://doi.org/10.1007/s10508-019-1397-6.

breathing with your partner if you're masturbating next to each other. It might feel challenging at the beginning but remember, we're not looking for perfection—just execution and follow-through.

Mixing different touches: If you have a go-to grip, toy, hand, or finger that you regularly use for masturbation, try something else. This practice is about being mindful and taking your time, but it's also about exploration. In our fast-paced world, we tend to rely on one thing and not put in extra effort to explore something new, whether it's a lunch spot, a TV show, or a way to masturbate. With mindful masturbation, I highly recommend mixing it up. I usually change the settings on or position of my vibrator to try a different sensation, or sometimes I'll use my fingers. For men, I recommend changing your grip, alternating your hand, and trying sex toys like a pocket pussy, stroker, or something else you prefer from the sexy shop. (I include recommended toys on my website, Luvbites.co, if you're unsure of where to start.)

Focusing on the now: Being present with your body is probably the hardest part of masturbation. Many people need porn stimulation when they masturbate, but for this exercise, you're not watching porn. Focusing on the now means you're just going to feel the sensations in your body, listen to your own breathing, and pat attention to the natural sounds of masturbation. There's no porn, no music, no external noise. If a random thought enters your mind, just accept it, let it go, and come back to focusing on your body.

Sexual Affirmations Through Journaling and Love Notes (Solo or Partnered)

This morning, I wrote in my journal, "I can feel my vagina intensely. I am proud of my body. I have amazing sexual energy." Yes, I believe in these statements wholeheartedly. I love the pleasurable feeling I experience when my vulva is properly stimulated. I love my body, even though it doesn't fit American beauty standards. And oh man, my sexual energy is off the charts. Of course I don't feel like that every day, but most days, I am a fucking *sex goddess*.

How did I get here? It hasn't always been like this, and journaling didn't heal my insecurities overnight. When I started daily journaling, I didn't believe a word I was writing, but I stuck with it and kept writing different positive sexual affirmations every day. After a couple months, my words started to feel authentic. What exactly are positive sexual affirmations? In short, they are positive and encouraging statements about our sexual self that we declare to be true. They can help us overcome shame, self-doubt, and negative thoughts about our sexuality. If you think, "I'm too anxious to have sex," then write, "I exude sexual confidence." If you feel ugly or physically undesirable, then write, "I am attractive and love my body." Over time, you can replace all the negative thoughts you have about your sex life, sexual desire, behaviors, and feelings with positive thoughts.

Why does it matter? Positive self-talk matters because it contributes to your empowerment and agency. Self-empowerment is one of the most important aspects of a healthy sex life—and, honestly, life as a whole. When you repeatedly write down and verbalize your affirmations, your brain actually changes. Neuroplasticity is the ability of neural networks in the brain to change and reorganize in response to learning, so it's definitely possible to "rewire" your cognitive pathways by telling your brain what to believe. That's why we should all do positive affirmations.

Sexual affirmation isn't just for self-talk, though. When it comes from a partner, it can also play a big role in enhancing your self-perceived attractiveness and sexual value. This can sound like, "OMG, I fucking love your body" or "You turn me on so much!" Partner affirmations matter because they express affection and admiration, which foster deeper connections and sexual self-esteem for both partners.

Here are five categories of affirmations. Feel free to use them in your daily life—or tweak them to your liking.

Body Love	• My body is a beautiful vessel for pleasure. • I love the way my body looks and feels. • I enjoy every part of my body.
Sexual Attitudes	• I'm empowered by my sexuality. • I embrace every aspect of my sexual self. • I appreciate my sexual thoughts and fantasies.
Sexual Behaviors	• I'm a great lover because I'm competent, mindful, and generous. • Good sex is amazing and is available to me. • Sexual exploration is fun and delightful.
Desired Outcomes for Self	• My body is filled with pleasurable sensations, and I can access them anytime I want. • When I have sex, it's passionate and enjoyable. • I can easily communicate my sexual desires and boundaries.
Desired Outcomes with Partner	• My partner and I have a great sex life. • My relationship is full of positive sexual energy. • My partner and I can easily communicate our sexual needs, desires, and issues.

VISUALIZATION (SOLO)

When was the last time you imagined yourself having the most passionate, highly connected, hot sex with insane chemistry? No, it doesn't have to be with your current partner. If you've never done it, or haven't done it recently, that's OK! That's what this exercise is all about: visualizing a successful sexual encounter. When you practice using your imagination, you'll find it easier to embody what you've imagined when it comes to real-life sexual situations. It's scientifically proven that imagined interactions have real-life effects[32]. So why not practice using your imagination? It's one of the best ways to practice sexual mindfulness—and best of all, it's free!

Start by closing your eyes or softly gazing somewhere. Every day can include a different type of visualization, but let's practice visualizing a successful sexual encounter. What type of sex are you craving right now? Is it slow and romantic? Heated and aggressive? Kinky and taboo? Maybe it's something that feeds your fantasies or a fetish. Whatever it is, I want you to think of one sexual encounter, a successful one that satiates you. Give as much context as possible.

Who are you interacting with? Is it just you? Who else is involved? What do they look like? Who are they? Is it your spouse, your partner, a random stranger, your neighbor? Lastly, think about the encounter itself. How does it start? Where are you? What does it look like? Are you inside or outside? In public or private? What is happening? Are you being dominated by someone or even a group of people? Are you initiating and taking control of the sex and your partner?

It doesn't have to stop at your imagination. You can record the situation for later consumption or to share with your partner(s). What do I mean? Record a voice note, record a video of you talking through it, or describe the visualization in your journal. Be as detailed as possible. Listen, watch, or read it again in a week or a month. Revisit it anytime you're curious for some mental stimulation.

Erotic Breathwork (Solo or Partnered)

Breath plays a *huge* role in sexual wellness in some specific ways. There is a direct, proven link between proper breathing and sexual function.

---

32. Joe Ayres and Brian L. Heuett, "An Examination of the Long-Term Effect of Performance Visualization," *Communication Research Reports* 17, no. 3 (2000): 229–236, https://doi.org/10.1080/08824090009388770.

Oxygen is essential for a healthy body, so improper breathing (e.g., mouth breathing[33] and consistent short breaths, which leads to a lack of oxygen) can lead to sexual dysfunctions such as erectile dysfunction, premature ejaculation, lack of sexual arousal, and low libido. By contrast, deep breathing exercises contribute to better blood flow to the genital area, which leads to better sexual functioning in both men and women. This is why I'm such a big proponent of regular breathwork.

There's an element of breathwork already embedded in sexual meditation, but the focus here is on erotic breathing. What's erotic breathing? It's a breathing exercise that fosters sexual mindfulness. You can do it by yourself as a self-care practice or with your partner as a couple's intimacy practice. Here are the steps:

1. **Take a deep breath in through your nose for as long as you can. For some people, that might be four seconds; for others, it might be ten seconds or more. Go at your own pace; this is not a competition.**

2. **Exhale through your mouth and let out an erotic moan (whatever that sounds like; it's all you). Make sure you breathe out all the way.**

3. **Take a deeper breath through the nose and focus on feeling the sensations in your sex organs while inhaling.**

4. **Exhale through your nose, emptying your lungs. As you do, your stomach will shrink.**

5. **Repeat steps 1–4. Beginners should start with five rounds (ten total breaths). If you have experience with breathwork, then try ten rounds (twenty total breaths). If you're up for a challenge, try fifteen rounds (thirty total breaths). You might even cum; I've done it before.**

If you're brand new to erotic breathing, I recommend trying for a seven-day streak. You'll see differences in yourself such as the ability

---

33. Amir Khalid Hassan, "Relation Between Mouth Breather Patients and Their Sexual Activities, Pilot Study," *Journal of Oral Health and Dental Science* 3, no. 2 (May 2019): 1-3.

to stay more present during sex, orgasm easier, and feel more pleasurable sensations. I always encourage people to do a small set daily because it's great for you, but if that's not your jam, try to embed it in your weekly routine. You can even start implementing this breathing technique during sex and see your orgasms intensify.

All the practices discussed in this chapter are research-based effective practices that can greatly enhance your sex life when you do them consistently. Just as you pay attention to your physical health at the gym, you also need to focus on your sexual well-being!

Chapter 4

Sex Student Honor's List: Sex Education for Adults

> ***Sex education is essential to create healthy self-knowledge and reconciliation, healthy conversation and understanding, healthy mindsets and lifestyles.***
>
> —Fatima Mohammed

Vulva or vagina? Grace didn't use the right term until she was thirty-eight, and she's not alone. Sexual knowledge is like financial freedom—everyone wants it, but it eludes many. Far too many people get their "sex education" from porn or their peers. (I don't know which is worse: listening to another high schooler for sex tips or having a grown man think a woman should be wet without foreplay). Consequently, plenty of people don't know a lot about sex despite a belief that "it should be natural instinct." We have sex and masturbate, so we're skilled, right? Well, no. But that's OK. It can change starting from today.

The world of sexual knowledge is *vast*. Have you ever seen a picture of Earth from the perspective of the Milky Way galaxy? That's, roughly speaking, how much most people actually know about sex and sexuality. As a sex professor, I still learn new things regularly. To be honest, it's impossible to teach a whole sex-ed course in one chapter, but I can give an overview of sexual knowledge so you can start your sexual awakening journey with confidence. So, in this chapter, I'll highlight different aspects of sexual knowledge to help you feel more sexually empowered. These aspects include self-concept, sexual and romantic orientations, sexual desire/sex drive, orgasms, sexual satisfaction, types of attraction, erogenous zones, and common issues.

Sexual knowledge falls into two categories: knowing more about yourself and knowing more about sex in general. Let's start with the first one because if you don't know who you are, then we don't know how to feed this sexy beast properly, right? Remember, in this book, I'm your sex professor, and I want you to make the honor roll.

SEXUAL SELF-CONCEPT

Sexual self-concept is how you perceive and describe your sexuality. If I ask you right now to take sixty seconds and write down five words that authentically and, in your opinion, accurately describe your sexuality, could you do it? Absolutely not? Don't know where to start? That's OK! That's the response I get from most people when I ask them to describe their sexual self. If you've read Chapter 1, you should be able to tell people your Sexual Profile, so that's a great start!

I'm a dynamic lover, which means I like mixing things up and trying new things. I'm kinky, so I'm down for some nontraditional stuff as long as we talk about it beforehand. (No stuffing food up my ass before consent!) I'm flexible when it comes to playing with others. I don't need to play in groups to experience pleasure, but once in a while , it can really spice things up and crank up that excitement factor. I'm an animalistic lover, which means I moan loudly and prefer intense sexual experiences, so quiet sex is hard for me and most likely won't turn me on. Apart from my sexual profile, another phrase that describes my self-concept is *sexually curious*. I'm always curious to know more about sex and what I would find enjoyable and not enjoyable.

Here are some sentence starters to help you describe your self-concept:

- **When I think of the sex I really enjoy, it usually includes an aspect of _______.**
- **When it comes to sex, I prefer _______.**
- **If I were my own lover, I would describe myself as _______.**

There are millions of ways to describe yourself, so feel free to grab a pen and paper and list as many things as you can! While this is a mainly solo activity, it's also a fun activity to do with your partner or during girl's night.

SEXUAL AND ROMANTIC ORIENTATIONS

There's more to sexual orientation than just straight or gay. Humans are complex. Scientists still don't have an explanation for why we experience certain thoughts, feelings, and emotions. We still don't understand consciousness, and like most human phenomena, sexual and romantic orientations are not black and white.

For example, I recently went to a dinner party and sat next to John. Through some open-minded conversation we shared that night, he told me his life story. He came out as gay when he was forty after being "in the closet" due to his family and cultural expectations. He said he never had the courage to come out for most of his life. He had a wife who was shocked but also understanding. After his divorce, he started dating men but noticed that he was still interested in having sex with some women, which caused confusion. I immediately and joyfully said, "Oh, it sounds like you're homoromantic and bisexual."

John's eyes widened as he said, "Homo what? I've never heard of that!" I pointed out that most people haven't heard of it, but I teach it in my college class about sexuality. After that conversation, I realized that these concepts are not widely known, despite them really helping people truly understand their identities.

"That makes so much sense!" John exclaimed. "I feel like I've unlocked a deeper understanding of myself and have language to share with people when they ask!" Our language represents our reality, so having accurate words that can authentically describe your personal identities can be life changing.

Your romantic orientation is who you're romantically attracted to and interested in. In other words, it's who you want to date or be in a romantic relationship with. You may be heteroromantic (romantically attracted to people of a different gender), homoromantic (romantically attracted to people of your own gender), biromantic (romantically attracted to men and women), panromantic (romantically interested in people of all genders), or aromantic (not romantically attracted to others).

By contrast, your sexual orientation is who you're attracted to sexually or want to have sex with. You may be heterosexual (sexually attracted to people of a different gender), homosexual (sexually attracted to people of the same gender), bisexual (sexually attracted to men and women), pansexual (sexually attracted to people of all genders), or asexual (not sexually attracted to others). Sometimes your romantic and sexual orientations align, such as if you're a lesbian and both sexually and romantically into women. You can enjoy dating a woman and having sex with her.

However, some people have mixed orientations, me included! I'm heteroromantic and bisexual, which means I'm romantically attracted to men (hence, I married my husband) and sexually attracted to both men and women (so I enjoy having recreational sex with both). Like I said, humans are complex, but language helps us understand ourselves and one another, so it's important to teach others and use accurate and descriptive language that helps you communicate with clarity. This should mitigate a lot of misunderstandings, confusion, and heartaches.

SEXUAL DESIRE/SEX DRIVE

When you're hungry, you need to eat. If you don't eat for a long time, you will die, so hunger is a biological need. However, if you don't have sex for a long time, you're not going to die (though you might feel otherwise if you haven't had sex in a long time). After all, you can still masturbate, gain pleasure, and get sexual relief. Yes, people's physical and mental health can be negatively affected by a lack of sexual connection, but you won't die as a result—so it's not necessarily a biological need. This is why some sexuality educators stopped teaching the term *sex drive* because it's just not that accurate. Many educators suggest that it's not a drive in the biological sense; it's a desire because you want it—but you don't need it.

Sexual desire is simply defined as the wish to engage in sexual activity. You can have high, moderate, or low sexual desire depending on your phase of life, the time of the month, your stress levels, and so many other factors. Your sexual desire is also dynamic. For instance, you might have high sexual desire in your early twenties (when you started to sexually explore and date other people) but you may experience low sexual desire after the death of a pet or after taking antidepressant medication for a while. You get the gist. There are various activities that can enhance your sexual desire (such as sexual meditation and regular self-pleasure sessions), but the most dangerous sexual-desire killer is stress. Therefore, if you want to increase your sexual desire, it's crucial to lower your stress level first.

Libido, in comparison, is a medical term for *sex drive*. Doctors may use the word *libido* to describe your sexual functioning. For example, a doctor may say, "Low testosterone can cause low libido." What about sexual urges? That's the same as libido; a sexual urge means wanting to have sex. Therefore, in a way, all these terms mean the same thing.

Sexual arousal, though, is different. Arousal is the feeling of being sexually turned on. When you're aroused, your body experiences physical and emotional responses. That can look like hardened nipples, an erect penis, or an erect clitoris (what I call "Clitosaurus"). Sexual *arousal* isn't the same thing as sexual *desire*. Have you ever felt horny but don't get wet or hard? That's because desire and arousal originate in different systems. Sometimes we have the desire (I'm horny!) but our body isn't responding fast enough (Why is my pussy not wet yet?). It's called arousal non-concordance, and it's *very* common. Longer foreplay and more exciting and sensual play will allow women time to get wet and men to get hard, so don't rush things—unless it's a quickie and that's what you want. I understand, not every meal needs to be at a Michelin star restaurant. Sometimes we just want fast food fries.

ORGASMS

Ahhhh! Orgasms are delicious. I absolutely love the feeling of orgasming. It's a rush of energy before a great release and, depending on the time of day, can lead to a really good sleep. Other times, orgasms give me more energy to make it through the day. It's important to remember, though, that an orgasm is peak sexual arousal but does not equate to sexual satisfaction and fulfillment. There are many types of orgasms and ways to orgasm.

Men can have an ejaculatory orgasm, which is the standard kind where you ejaculate from the penis. A pelvic orgasm is where you orgasm through edging but don't ejaculate. A prostate orgasm (p-spot) is where you orgasm from getting your prostate stimulated. The prostate is located about two inches inside the butt hole, so don't be shy about putting a pinky inside if you want to start exploring the p-spot orgasm (with consent, of course). A testical orgasm (ballgasm) is a fun one where you orgasm from getting your balls stimulated. Technically, men can have multiple orgasms when they fully explore their body. Ejaculation is just one of several ways.

Women can also experience many types of orgasms. A clitoral orgasm (yum!) is the easiest to access for most women. It comes from repeatedly stimulating the clitoris, which has over ten thousand nerve endings and its sole purpose is to give you pleasure. A vaginal orgasm is the pleasurable feeling from inside the vagina overall—caused by stimulation to the clitoral network and its thousands of nerve endings. A g-spot orgasm comes from stimulating the g-spot, which is located a few inches inside the vagina on top of the vaginal canal. Some women have never experienced this despite many attempts, so you'll often hear certain people say the g-spot is a myth. (I'll let you decide for yourself.) A cervical orgasm (c-spot) is accessed by stimulating deep inside the vagina—by massaging and stimulating the cervical area. Not all women like their c-spot stimulated; in fact, many say it can be painful, so, again, to each their own. A squirting orgasm is when you ejaculate fluids at the moment of climax. Some women squirt a lot, some only a little. There are many methods to get there, but many women (myself included) have enjoyed squirting orgasms via being fingered. There are many fingering techniques, but the most common one is the "come hither" motion with one or two fingers. There isn't agreement among researchers whether this fluid is urine. Most sex specialists will tell you it's a mix of different fluids that come mostly from the Skene's glands. I say just enjoy it and don't worry so much about where it's from.

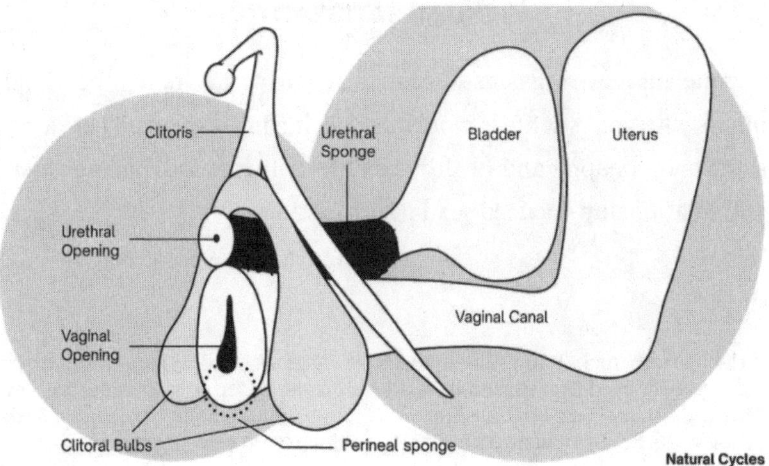

In addition, there are many other types of orgasms that are available for everyone to experience. Nipple orgasms come from nipple stimulation. Coregasms can be accessed through different types of exercise that stimulate your body. To be honest, I've never experienced this one, but I look forward to having it one day (going back to my crunches now). Interestingly, a national survey[34] of sexual health and behavior in 2014 showed that 9 percent of respondents experienced an exercise-induced orgasm. Blended orgasms are when you orgasm from different areas at the same time. For women, the most common case would be having simultaneous clitoral and vaginal orgasms; for men, it would be ejaculation via anal play. Anal orgasms are another type that both men and women can experience. I'll tell you a secret: I've never had an anal orgasm, but many people have and find it enjoyable.

Here's a summary for everyone who loves lists:

Men	Women	Everyone
Ejaculatory orgasm	Clitoral orgasm	Nipple orgasm
Pelvic orgasm	Vaginal orgasm	Coregasm
Prostate orgasm	G-spot orgasm	Blended orgasm
Testicle orgasm	Cervical orgasm	Anal orgasm

SEXUAL SATISFACTION

As much as I love orgasms—because they're great—remember that happiness with your sex life is more than just having orgasms. There are three aspects to a happy and healthy sex life: self-focused, partner-focused, and relationship-focused sexual satisfaction.

34. Debby Herbenick, Tsung-Chieh Fu, Callie Patterson, and J. Dennis Fortenberry, "Exercise-Induced Orgasm and Its Association with Sleep Orgasms and Orgasms During Partnered Sex: Findings from a U.S. Probability Survey," *Archives of Sexual Behavior* 50, no. 6 (August 2021): 2631–2640, doi: 10.1007/s10508-021-01996-9.

For self-focused sexual satisfaction, it's all about you. Are you happy with your sexual functioning, sexual arousal, and sexual desire levels? How do you feel about your ability to let go and feel all the pleasure during sex? Do you experience shame, guilt, or anxiety? Are you happy with the way you're able to engage in sexual encounters? How do you feel about your experiences of orgasms?

For partner-focused sexual satisfaction, it's all about your partner(s). Are they a good and generous lover to you? Do they contribute to your pleasure in a significant way? How do you feel about the way they have sex with you? Are there a lot of things you want your partner to change when it comes to sex, or do you feel pretty in sync with each other? Are you happy with your partner's sexual functioning, sexual arousal, and sexual desire levels?

For relationship-focused sexual satisfaction, it's all about the interpersonal communication between the two (or more) of you. Are you able to have an open-minded conversation about sex together? Do you feel judged or accepted by your partner? How do you feel about your interactions when it comes to sex? Does your sexual relationship bring you some type of joy or happiness? Are you able to communicate your sexual concerns and interests without fear?

Being sexually satisfied is an amazing feeling and contributes positively to every aspect of your life. Sexual fulfillment, by contrast, is like the mother of sexual satisfaction. If you rate your sex life 7 out of 10, you're satisfied. A truly fulfilling sex life, though, merits a 10 out of 10 rating. You can be satisfied with your current situation but still be curious and want to explore other sexual experiences or want to make your current sexual relationship even more passionate and energetically aligned. Sexual fulfillment is dynamic. Maybe you feel sexually fulfilled in March but not in May. It takes effort and sometimes we don't prioritize our sex life due to other obligations—and that's fine. Just know that you can always do the exercises in this book to enhance your sex life and achieve your own version of sexual fulfillment. A fulfilling sex life is 100 percent within reach for everyone.

TYPES OF ATTRACTION

What are you into? A big part of knowing your sexual self is knowing what's attractive to you. When you're attracted to someone or the specific ways they do things (or even to certain personal traits, such as the way they smell), sexual arousal and enjoyment comes a lot easier.

I've found that people who are more sexually satisfied find their partners attractive in their own way. Right now, rate your partner's (or the person you're casually dating) attractiveness on a scale from 1 to 10—and be honest! Do you think that affects your motivation to have sex with them? Hell yeah it does! It definitely plays a role in your sexual desire. Almost everyone has a favorite thing about their sexual partner that they're extremely attracted to. This can be anything from physical characteristics (like broad shoulders or nice legs), a certain way they express their personality (like confidence, sarcasm, or goofiness), or some type of competence that's appealing (like that they own their business or are a talented artist). So let's explore your perception of attraction and attractiveness together.

Physical attraction: Although some people claim they don't care about physical attractiveness, research[35] has revealed that it actually matters—but not in a way we might think. Yes, there are attractiveness theories that state certain qualities are perceived as more attractive. For example, the facial symmetrical theory says that people are generally

[35] Adrian Furnham et al., "Waist to Hip Ratio and Facial Attractiveness: A Pilot Study," *Personality and Individual Differences* 30, no. 3 (February 2001): 491–502, https://doi.org/10.1016/s0191-8869(00)00040-4.

perceived as more attractive when their face is symmetrical. The hip-to-waist ratio theory says that when your hips are 1.5 times your waist, then you're more likely to be seen as attractive. Do these rules apply in every situation? Not really. As they say, beauty is in the eye of the beholder and there are plenty of people around the world who do not meet these "standards" and are still perceived as attractive by many. One of the physical characteristics that I find *very hot* is long hair. Yes, I have a thing for guys with long hair. Not all of them, of course, but it's the extra *umph* for me. What about you? What physical characteristics do you find particularly attractive?

Social attraction: Aren't some people just so damn charismatic? One of the most valued types of attractiveness is a good personality. People often say, "Oh, I don't care about looks; I care more about personality." OK, but what personality? Are you able to identify qualities that you find attractive? Do you prefer someone who is refined and sophisticated or rougher around the edges and simple? Do you prefer someone who is talkative and outgoing or quieter and more observant? Do you prefer someone who is bold and assertive or a bit more passive and agreeable? Knowing more about your preferences can help you manifest and attract the right person for you—and even point out if the person you're dating is compatible with you or not.

Sexual attraction: This is like having sex appeal or sexual chemistry with someone. It's attraction on the basis of sexual desire. You can be attracted to someone because you want to be friends with them and don't find them sexually attractive. Physical appearance influences sexual attraction, but so do many other factors, such as what it feels like when they touch and kiss you and what they smell, taste, or sound like. Someone's movement can also contribute to sexual attractiveness. Do you like the way they walk, dance, or move their hips? Some people claim sexual attraction isn't important when it comes to finding a long-term partner. For me, though? It's *very* important!

Intellectual attraction: Have you ever talked to someone about something meaningful and, wow, you just feel a mental connection? That's most likely because you find them intellectually attractive. Some people have certain knowledge about the world, a certain industry, or unfamiliar human experiences, and you just find yourself being drawn toward them. You're attracted to their thoughts, the way they have conversations, their worldview, their knowledge, their wisdom. Personally, I don't know too much about world history, so I find people who know a lot about history very attractive. What is an intellectual quality you find attractive?

Spiritual attraction: A strong spiritual connection is hard to describe. It's when you're drawn to someone's energy. You find them powerful and attractive without particular physical-world attributes. A spiritual connection exists on a deeper level. You might be initially drawn to someone's energy and then develop a spiritual attraction through conversations with them. It's not necessarily that you share a religion or practice the same faith (although that can play a role). You can find someone attractive when you're interested in their spirituality, you feel safe and comfortable around them, you feel like there's synchronicity between you, and you feel strong empathy for each other.

EROGENOUS ZONES

Stephanie loves it when her husband eats her ass. In this case, Steph's anus is one of her active erogenous zones. An erogenous zone is an area of your body that brings pleasurable feelings when stimulated, which contributes to your sexual arousal. The obvious ones are lips, nipples, and genitals, but we actually have more than twenty erogenous zones! It depends on whether or not it's an active zone. What does that mean? Well, we're all wired differently. Steph may get aroused by having her bootyhole played with, but other people might not because it's not an active zone for them. Is it possible to activate the zone? Sure, you can, but only if you really want to! Sensation mapping exercises can help you activate/reactivate certain areas of your body that can bring a lot of pleasure. You won't know if a certain body part can bring pleasure to you unless you've tried to stimulate it.

Mike had nipple play hesitation for a long time. He wasn't able to receive pleasure from having his nipples licked or massaged, but he wanted to, so he embarked on a sexual exploration journey through a sensation mapping exercise. This exercise can be done by yourself, with a partner, or with a somatic sex coach/therapist. (I need to note that many people have reported it's easier to do this exercise with a partner because touching yourself versus being touched can be a totally different experience). Sensation mapping involves using different types of touch on different areas of the body, particularly the erogenous zones. The three types of touch are soft touch, passionate touch (stronger grip), and dominant touch (strongest grip). As you go through your body's different erogenous zones, try a soft touch for sixty seconds and then tell your partner if you want to try a passionate touch or move on to a different area. Here's a list of the erogenous zones. Have fun!

Erogenous Zones

- **Scalp**
- **Lips**
- **Ears**
- **Neck**
- **Nipples**
- **Lower back**
- **Inner arms**

- **Abs**
- **Pubic area**
- **Butt cheeks**
- **Butthole**
- **Genital area**
- **Inner thighs**
- **Calves**
- **Feet**

COMMON ISSUES

How do you build and rebuild sexual intimacy?

I completely trust that my husband loves me and wants me to experience pleasure, that he cares about my wellness (including sexual wellness), that I can tell him my sexual fantasies and exploration without being judged, and that I can let go during sex and feel all of the delicious sensations. This is possible because we've built and continuously maintained our sexual intimacy. Building sexual intimacy isn't about having sex every day. It comes from a combination of physical closeness, emotional closeness, and trust. When you lack one part of the equation, you might feel like your relationship is "out of sync." When it comes to sexual intimacy, many men tend to focus on physical closeness and neglect emotional closeness. On the other hand, I've seen a lot of women who crave emotional closeness but neglect physical closeness. Trust is also an extremely important part of the formula. Do you trust that your partner has your best interests at heart? Do you trust that they care about you, your feelings and emotions, your physical and mental health, and your sexual well-being? To build this trust and intimacy, you have to consistently practice nonjudgmental communication.

Whenever you express judgment to your partner, they lose a bit of trust in you. In addition, you both feel less intimate, so empathetic communication is vital in a sexually intimate relationship. Another factor is consistency. Do you walk the walk or just talk the talk? If you say you want to pleasure your partner but don't listen to their feedback, that inconsistency reduces trust in your relationship. Follow-through is how you gain trust. When your partner does what they say they'll do, it allows you to feel safe and relaxed—like you can truly trust them. Of course, physical intimacy (regular sexual activity) is an important part of sexual intimacy. In short, couples feel closer together when they're sexually satisfied and fulfilled. What that looks like, however, is different for every couple. Some couples are happy with sex a few times a week, a month, or even a year. It's up to you, but you have to communicate your expectations to each other. That's how you build sexual intimacy.

Most couples find they are sexually satisfied and feel sexually intimate within the first few years of the relationship. What happens after a few years? Well, it's common to hear that the relationship lacks spark, passion, or sexual intimacy. This is because that spark comes from novelty and excitement. At a certain point in any relationship, the spark should no longer be your sexual goal because it's unrealistic and unproductive. You're not the same person you were a few years ago, and your relationship developed so much in that time. Therefore, it's time to set a new sexual goal together. Maybe it's an exciting exploration into nontraditional sex or tantric sex. Maybe it's trying sexual meditation or sexological bodywork. Maybe it's going to a nudist resort for fun. Whatever you decide, the key is to keep a curious mindset as you sexplore new territory together. Rebuilding your sexual intimacy can look like setting new sexual goals, having regular conversations about sexual well-being, and following through with what you talked about. Remember, your sex life can get better when you put in the effort.

I'm singling and mingling. Should I have sex on the first date if the chemistry is there?

This is actually a controversial topic, and there's no right or wrong answer for this one. It depends on what school of thought you subscribe to and the person you're on a date with. People who enjoy sex on the first date are often called so many unkind things: whore, slut, asshole, douchebag . . . you get the idea. But why do we need to penalize people for basically just going for what they want? Lots of internet gurus say you should wait to "prove your value" or that a woman is not "wife material" if she sleeps with you on the first date. It's all misogynistic bullshit. Anyone can and should enjoy sex the way they want to as long as it's between consenting adults. Still, there is plenty of misunderstanding about this topic.

There are two schools of thought: sexual restraint and sexual compatibility. If you subscribe to the former, you're someone who would never have sex on the first date regardless of how amazing it went, how much chemistry there was, or how much you want to fuck the other person. You don't enjoy sex with someone if there's no emotional intimacy between you, so you'd rather wait and see how the relationship develops. After trust has grown and you feel emotionally connected to each other, then you'll fuck them.

The other side of that coin is the sexual compatibility model. If you subscribe to this school, then you're more likely to have sex on the first date if it goes well and there's chemistry because you want to know right away if you are sexually compatible. If sexual compatibility is crucial to a good relationship, then yeah, you'll want to find out as soon as possible. At the end of the day, the world is a better place when we communicate what we want and why we want it and when we can respect other people's choices without putting them down.

What can we do if we have mismatched sexual desires?

This is so common. Have you ever felt like you want more sex than your partner does, or vice versa? I've been in a relationship where my partner rarely initiated sex with me (like once every three months or so), and it was not good for me. It took a toll on my confidence and overall energy. Even though I was masturbating regularly, I became sexually frustrated—which grew into a general frustration with him and so much of what he did. Even after a conversation about trying harder in our sex life, nothing changed. I didn't blame him because it wasn't his fault. We were sexually incompatible and should have had the conversation—and parted ways—much earlier in the relationship. He didn't think sex was important in a long-term relationship, which is the opposite of what I believe. This is just one example of so many stories about mismatched sexual desires.

The first thing you'll have to do is have a proper conversation about the situation with your partner. Some people are able to compromise and have a healthy sex life, but nothing can be fixed unless both partners admit to the current struggle and commit to changing for the better. You can have this conversation by yourselves in private or have it with a sex coach/therapist; a professional third party can often help you navigate this difficult conversation. Remember, you're not alone in this struggle. It's one of the most common issues that long-term couples experience. For the big convo, here are some questions to ask and answer:

- **How would you rate our sex life, from 1 to 10, this past year? Why?**
- **What are some things I can do more or less of to help us have better sex?**
- **What are some things you want to do more or less of to help us have better sex?**
- **What are some things you want to explore sexually next year?**
- **How important is our sexual well-being, on a scale from 1 to 10? Why?**
- **What do you think should be our new sexual goals?**

The answers to these questions should uncover some truths about what's going on in your sex life. Ultimately, there are three potential outcomes: 1) You compromise and work together to meet and maintain your sexual goals, 2) you realize that you're sexually incompatible and then decide whether that's a dealbreaker for your relationship, or 3) you find creative solutions to the situation.

Here are some examples of sexual goals. These are actual goals that I helped my clients create, based on their desires:

- **We will find time to be sexually intimate at least once a week. We will turn our phones off and put in the effort to have a satisfying sex session.**
- **We will explore two sex clubs this year. The goal isn't to have sex with other people (we're not ready yet) but to expose ourselves to new erotic experiences.**
- **We will try BDSM practices at home once a month. We will be mindful about learning ethical BDSM together by taking an online class and enacting what we learn.**
- **We will try sexting each other at least once a week to spice things up. We will find creative ways to sext.**
- **We will do daily sexual meditation together for at least three months.**
- **We will give each other oral sex at least once a week.**
- **We will go sex toy shopping once every three months and use that toy to sexually explore.**
- **We will masturbate together once a week and watch each other masturbate once a month.**
- **We will try going to a nudist resort for fun this year.**
- **We promise to stay present and committed every time we have sex.**

These are just a few examples. Feel free to create your own, based on your interests and desires. Everyone is different and we all want different things, but, ultimately, most of us want a good sex life. Share your desires with your partner so you can work together toward making them a reality. The quality of your sex life is in your own hands.

How does your attachment style affect your dating and sexual behaviors?

Frank has an avoidant attachment style, so after having sex with Chloe on their second date, he didn't think to text her until three days had passed. At that point, Chloe felt like he was not actually interested in having a serious relationship, so she moved on and started swiping on dating apps again. Our attachment style exhibits itself in our dating and sexual behaviors—sometimes in a good way, sometimes disastrous.

There are four attachment styles: secure, anxious, avoidant, and disorganized. A secure attachment means you have a positive view of yourself and others. You trust your partner. You feel that you can rely on them, and vice versa. You are able to have a healthy interdependent relationship. It's like "You're cool, I'm cool, we're cool!" An anxious attachment means you have a positive view of your partner but a negative view of yourself. You struggle with self-esteem and have a deep fear of abandonment. You sometimes think that your partner is going to leave you. You need a lot of affirmations and attention from your partner. It's like "Oh no, they haven't texted me in five hours, they must not love me!" An avoidant attachment means you have a positive view of yourself but a negative view of others. It's hard for you to give someone a lot of time and effort. You can't fully trust others so you don't want to rely on them and don't want them to rely on you. It's like "I don't need anybody! I'm good on my own!" A disorganized attachment means you struggle over bonding with someone. Sometimes you feel like you need space, but other times you want your partner to be with you 24/7. You have a deep fear of getting hurt, and your partner and your relationship cause you both fear and desire. It's like "I love them, but they haven't said they love me yet, so maybe I'll dump them before they dump me. Bye!"

Yes, your attachment style influences your sexual attitudes and behaviors. For example,

- **People with an insecure attachment may use sex as a remedy in their own way. For example, an anxious person may use sex as a way to feel romantically affirmed and more connected with their sexual partner whether or not they actually wanted to have sex or enjoyed the sex itself. What matters is that they feel like their partner still wants them.**
- **An avoidant person may use sex for pleasure without properly communicating to their sexual partner whether they have romantic intentions because that conversation might be a burden. They also don't usually engage in affectionate foreplay.**
- **A disorganized person may confuse sex as a way their sexual partner communicates affection. They feel unworthy of love and sexual pleasure and often use casual sex as a way to avoid getting too close to anybody.**
- **A secure person enjoys sex for pleasure and for developing and maintaining a connection with their partner.**

What's the point of knowing all this? Well, I think it's a great start for your healing journey. If you identify as one of the insecure attachment styles, you can look into various methods of healing and growth so you can develop a secure attachment with your current or future partner. My friend Dr. Morgan Anderson is an attachment style expert and has lots of helpful resources. Check her out! Learning about your and your partner's attachment style is a journey, so be patient, open-minded, and willing to learn and communicate.

DR. TARA'S RELATIONAL IDENTITY EXERCISE

This short exercise can help clarify your relational identity and give you proper language to talk about yourself and what you're into!

I am romantically interested in dating . . .

- **Women**
- **Trans women**
- **Men**
- **Trans men**
- **Men and women**
- **Anyone (When it comes to dating, I don't think about gender.)**

I am sexually interested in having sex with . . .

- **Women**
- **Trans women**
- **Men**
- **Trans men**
- **Men and women**
- **Anyone (When it comes to sex, I don't think about gender.)**

SEXUAL KNOWLEDGE REPORT CARD

Do some self-reflection and rate your current sexual knowledge (1–10), then write down the goal that you want to get to next year. For example, foreplay = 6, next year = 8.

Sexual knowledge	Current Rating	Desired Rating
Knowing your SEXUAL SELF-CONCEPT		
Knowing your ROMANTIC and SEXUAL ORIENTATION		
Knowing different types of ATTRACTION and ATTRACTIVENESS		
Understanding LIBIDO and SEXUAL DESIRE		
Understanding EROGENOUS ZONES		
Understanding FOREPLAY		
Skills for INTERCOURSE		
Understanding different types of ORGASMS		
Knowing your ATTACHMENT STYLE		
Understanding how to build SEXUAL INTIMACY		

My goal with this chapter was to provide you with foundational knowledge to set you up for a fulfilling sex life. Of course, sexual wellness consists of much more than one chapter of words, but I hope that it inspires you to read the rest of the book with enthusiasm and provokes you to further explore the world of sexuality in your own way! Let's all change the world for the better, one sex-positive person at a time!

Chapter 5

No Kink Shaming Allowed: Nontraditional Sexual Behavior

If it is the dirty element that gives pleasure to the act of lust, then the dirtier it is, the more pleasurable it is bound to be.

—Marquis de Sade

John and Brenda have been together for three years. For the first two years, they had what most people call "vanilla sex." It's the term used to describe sexual activities that are considered conventional for adults, typically exemplified by missionary sex in bed with dimmed lights. It starts with conventional foreplay—like kissing and maybe oral—then penetration, and finally orgasm (hopefully for all parties involved, but statistically that's not the case). Let me be clear, there is *no vanilla shaming* here. In fact, that sex I just described sounds perfectly divine and pleasurable as long as the lovers are really into it. But Brenda, after dating for three years, realized that John loves food play because he keeps asking her to participate in it. No, he doesn't just *enjoy* food play or think about it from time to time—it's actually one of his kinks. He sexually desires food play more than anything else but has been suppressing his desires because he didn't want to be judged negatively.

After a few years of being together in a loving relationship, he felt comfortable and safe that Brenda would love and accept him for who he is, so he started sharing more and more of his kink. The act that he really loves, and that turns him on so much, is using whipped cream during sex. Specifically, he loves putting whipped cream on her pussy as he goes to town eating her pussy passionately. But lately, he's been asking to shoot whipped cream up Brenda's ass then have her push it out as he observes and jerks himself off.

Brenda is concerned. Is John sick? Does he have issues? Should he see a doctor so he can find treatment for this perversion? Nope, John's fine. Unless he's psychologically afflicted otherwise, there's nothing wrong with food play as a sexual kink. This sexual act may make a lot of us uncomfortable or even disgusted because it's socially taboo and unconventional. If it's not your thing, then it's not your thing, but millions of people around the world enjoy unconventional sex. My general good rule of thumb is as long as it's *legal, consensual, and pleasurable*, it's all good. Don't yuck other people's yum. Everyone is allowed to have their own sexual imagination, and they're allowed to act it out if they want to.

In John and Brenda's case, it's not the act that's bad—it's the lack of proper communication on both sides. John needed to properly communicate his desires up front with Brenda so they could both plan for food play together, instead of bringing it up during sex and trying to act it out then and there. As a result, Brenda was uncomfortable and concerned because she didn't understand it. The good thing is they were able to meet with a sex coach who helped them understand the situation and communicate more clearly and intentionally. This chapter explores different kinks and fetishes in an accessible and humorous way. There's so much kink shaming in the world. It's time to bust balls and start to understand different kinks. No, you're not mentally ill if you enjoy BDSM. No, you're not needy if you have a praise kink. Yes, you're certified spicy if you enjoy spanking!

WHAT MAKES SOMETHING TABOO?

What makes certain sexual activities taboo while others are acceptable? In short, taboo sex is any sexual activity that's not deemed "normal" by mainstream culture, which is in turn determined by the dominant group of people in that culture. In Thailand (where I grew up), people put their palms together and bow to say hello. In France, they kiss each other on the cheek. If you do that in Thailand, especially between younger and older people, it would be considered weird and, dare I say, taboo, because it's not normal.

Culture, religion, and media create and reinforce the list of norms. Being gay used to be a crime in parts of the United States (it's not anymore), and it is still taboo and illegal in many countries and cultures around the world. Divorce used to be extremely taboo, but now it's normal. In some subcultures such as Mormonism, vaginal sex is not accepted but inserting the penis inside the vagina is fine as long as you're not moving or thrusting (it's called *soaking*). What's considered "normal" is very subjective. One person's normal is someone else's weird. But when it comes to sex, people can get extremely judgmental toward others who enjoy nontraditional things. That's partially because they fear what's different and because it's easier to judge than try to understand.

The media also plays a big part in the normalization of behaviors. What we see on TV and in movies influences our perceptions. For example, the movie *Fifty Shades of Grey* (love it or hate it) spiked an interest in practicing and more acceptance of BDSM relationships and activities. (I must acknowledge that some BDSM practitioners have issues with this movie's representation of real BDSM.) Social media also plays a role in how certain sexual acts are deemed "normal" or "gross." As a part of the lecture I give about online sex work, I show my students the websites where people submit photos of their feet and get paid.

I had a student who said, "Eww, that's gross. I'd never date a guy who's into feet."

I then asked, "What if he's perfect in every way for you and you really like him?"

She responded, "Nah, I can't get past the feet thing." Well, who you choose to date is up to you, but the unfortunate essence of that statement is that the person is judged by his sexual interests in feet. This is why most people find it hard to "come out of the closet" with their nontraditional sexual interests. The world would be a much better place if we could all be more compassionate and tolerant toward one another's preferences and differences. What's taboo is merely a difference in attitude and behavior.

WHY IS TABOO SEX SO EXCITING?

I believe we all have a little rebellious energy in us that can be exhibited in different ways. For some, it might be getting a tattoo, going bungee jumping, or racing cars, whereas for others, it might be having a threesome, watching other people have sex, having people watch you get flogged, being told you can't cum, licking honey off someone's butthole, or role-playing as professor and student. The list goes on and on. Prohibition didn't stop people from drinking, and abstinence-only sex education didn't stop people from having sex. People have always done things they "weren't supposed to do."

Our ancient ancestors used to have to run away from wild animals to save themselves and their family. For them, many days were full of adrenaline and life-and-death matters. Nowadays, though, many of us work monotonous jobs with a lot of stability—but also boredom. We come home, sit on the couch, and binge a Netflix show for hours. For some, life has become *too* comfortable and predictable. Let's be real: The modern rules-dominated world has led to some of us becoming deadly bored, and we long for sexual escapes—if for no other reason than to provide a change of pace in our lives. Taboo sex can serve as the adrenaline rush factor we desire, and going against the norm can satisfy that rebellious energy in ways you cannot do in your life outside sex.

I should note that I'm not an expert in these kinks and fetishes. Expertise requires a deep understanding of human behavior, history, and sexual psychology. If you're interested, there are ethical practitioners or experts in almost every kink and fetish you can contact and learn more from. The trick is to learn from the people with hands-on knowledge and experience (i.e., people who actually engage with the kinks and fetishes) and not just people who only talk about them. For example, learning about domination from a professor (like me) would give you a rudimentary understanding, but learning from a professional dominatrix who has been in the industry for more than ten years would provide a richer and more thorough understanding. Remember that sex educators teach concepts and normalize sexual behaviors (to reduce shame in the world of consensual sex and pleasure) but are not necessarily experts in everything.

KINKS VERSUS FETISHES

Kink is a broad term that's used to describe unconventional sexual acts and interests. Kinky sex consists of hundreds—if not thousands—of sexual activities, some more popular and practiced than others. People who practice kinky sex are called *kinksters*. Most kinks present no danger to the kinksters; on the other hand, some can be dangerous (but that's often the point of those types of kinks) and must be practiced with extreme caution (e.g., breath play, needle play). When someone has a fetish, they find it very difficult to achieve arousal and pleasure without that fetish being present or addressed. For someone with a foot fetish, for example, feet are a necessary arousal factor in their sexual encounters. There's some overlap between kinks and fetishes, but, overall, I find *kink* is the easiest term to use because it encompasses all unconventional sex. Not all kinksters are good or bad, just like not all pastors and priests are good or bad. Some kinksters practice their kinks ethically and carefully, but some bad apples are just . . . well, terrible people exist everywhere. People have had kinks and fetishes forever; this is not a new phenomenon.

Even though kinky sex has always been practiced, it's usually done behind closed doors, so there hasn't been a lot of proper documentation aside from rumors, stories, and cave drawings. There were stories of men having sex with animals in ancient Egypt (i.e., bestiality, which is illegal now and not condoned), group sex in ancient Greece, and boat orgies with Roman Emperor Caligula. There are violent sex paintings from the Middle Ages. And of course there's the rumor that Cleopatra had a vibrator (a phallic-shaped object filled with live bees). One of the earliest documented references to kinky sex is the *Kama Sutra*, which is estimated to be thousands of years old.

Psychologists have been studying kinks and fetishes for many years. Most kinks are harmless, but some kinks and fetishes can be harmful, such as those that inflict excessive pain in themselves with no boundaries. A fetishistic disorder[36] is when someone's fetish becomes a barrier for that person to have a productive life. It may cause extreme stress or dysfunction in work, relationships, and daily activities. When a kink becomes a disorder, it's best for the person to reach out to a sex therapist to work through their situation. On the other hand, if you like wearing leather outfits and enjoy engaging in power play as a dom or sub in your free time, there's nothing wrong with that. Have fun!

TWELVE POPULAR KINKS AND FETISHES

Role-play: Lots of kinky lovers enjoy role-play because it allows them to put their imaginations into practice and helps them overcome their inhibitions. Imagine being a sexy, naughty, and very bad patient trying to seduce a hot and unethical doctor to have totally taboo sex with you.

36. Antonio Ventriglio et al., "Sexuality in the 21st Century: Leather or Rubber? Fetishism Explained," *Medical Journal Armed Forces India* 75, no. 2 (April 2019): 121–124, https://doi.org/10.1016/j.mjafi.2018.09.009.

Sound like fun? If you're into that or other ideas that involve acting out a scene of taboo sex, then you're into role-play. The great thing about role-play is that the ideas are endless, and it can be as intense or chill as you desire. It can be a student having sex with a teacher, a boss ordering her employee to eat her pussy, or a yoga instructor groping a student in class. Want to get in the car and pretend to be a taxi driver getting a blowjob from a hot passenger? You can do it. Want to act like you're asleep when a robber is trying to have sex with you? Absolutely. Want to pretend to be a vampire and have "forced" sex with a human? You sure can. Also, who says you have to be human? Alien sex is apparently a popular fantasy as evidenced by the prevalence of alien porn on major porn sites. There's so much possibility with role-playing, but remember, it must be consensual by all parties involved. It's also more fun when everyone is into it.

Foot fetish: This is by far the most common fetish in the world[37]. There are countless online groups for foot lovers, it's one of the most popular porn genres, and there are multiple websites that serve millions of users with foot fetishes. A foot fetish isn't as simple as looking at any feet, though. There's a misconception that people with this fetish can just go to the beach, look at all the feet, and get aroused. It's not that simple. Many people with foot fetishes enjoy playing with feet while being stimulated sexually. Some people gain sexual gratification by getting stepped on by women wearing stilettos. Some people love feet in socks or stockings. Either way, it doesn't matter. As long as it doesn't hurt anybody, there's no shame in the foot fetish game. Communicate your desires up front, and people who are meant for you will understand you. Hopefully, with this book and the rise of sex positivity around the world, there will be fewer judgmental people and more sex-positive people.

Praise kink: "It makes me feel so sexy and confident, like an alluring sex queen, when he praises me," said Jenn. Her favorite praise? "You look

---

37. C. Scorolli et al., "Relative Prevalence of Different Fetishes," *International Journal of Impotence Research* 19, no. 4 (February 2007): 432–437, https://doi.org/10.1038/sj.ijir.3901547.

so fucking beautiful when you suck my cock" and "you're such a good girl." Isn't that so hot? Still, I know it's not for everybody. Some people are uncomfortable with overt praise in bed; it's a turn-off for them, and that's OK—it's a kink for a reason. I definitely have praise kink. It's the combination of verbal aggression and compliments that gets me. Having a praise kink is very common. In fact, if you search #praisekink on TikTok, you'll find over 90 million views—yeah, Gen Z has normalized this one. Is it because we constantly need validation? Not necessarily. Although a few people may need this purely because of their need for external validation, most people just find it's their preferred love language. A common love language is an affirmation in itself, so it's totally OK if you desire the same thing in bed. For example, my husband says "I love you so much" before he goes to work (which makes me feel happy, warm, and fuzzy) and then says "You're such a good girl for daddy" during sex (which makes me feel aroused and horny). Another benefit is that we get a rush of dopamine when we're complimented[38] (and when we give compliments), so it makes both lovers feel good and relaxed. There are many ways people can give compliments in bed for their partners who have a praise kink. It's best to ask them what phrases really turn them on, so ask, "Hey babe, what kind of praises do you like to hear in bed? What really turns you on?" The trick is to practice saying it by yourself in private so you gain fluency and confidence through practice. Then, during sex, you can feel more confident as you give your praises with conviction. Praises don't have to be aggressive. Some like it gentle, like "You're doing such a good job baby," whereas others may like "You're doing a great job, my little slut." You know . . . preferences.

Humiliation and degradation: "Your dick is so fucking small. It disgusts me!" Did that turn you on? Either it's the idea of saying it or receiving it, if it did, then you may have a small penis humiliation

[38]. Monica Eckstein, Gabriela Stößel, Martin Fungisai Gerchen, Edda Bilek, Peter Kirsch, and Beate Ditzen, "Neural Responses to Instructed Positive Couple Interaction: An fMRI Study of Compliment Sharing," *Social Cognitive and Affective Neuroscience* 18, no. 1 (February 2023), doi: 10.1093/scan/nsad005.

kink. The world of humiliation is vast, believe it or not. Many people enjoy verbal humiliation (e.g., being called names, degrading terms, or belittling phrases), whereas others may enjoy physical humiliation and degradation (e.g., being forced to kneel down). There are also quite a few tools commonly used in a humiliation kink (e.g., using a chastity device to lock up the genitalia is a way to humiliate and degrade erotically). Physical humiliation may also involve (consensual) forced oral, vaginal, and anal sex. Other impact play, such as slapping, may be included in a humiliation and degradation kink. Peeing on someone, using them as furniture, sitting on someone's face, forcing them to do things like eating without utensils, or having them kneel down before you or bow when you enter the room is also a part of this kink. Yes, this is a part of BDSM and power play overall, but it also is its own type of kink. Common humiliating words and phrases include *bitch, slut, stupid whore, you're worthless, Is this the best you can do?, You should be ashamed of your body, You're a piece of shit, You're nothing, Are you even in? I can't feel it, Your ___ is disgusting*, and *Shut your dirty mouth*. Isn't this just dirty talk? Well, yes and no. Humiliation is a category of dirty talk, but dirty talk in general doesn't have to be degrading or humiliating—it can be quite loving. By contrast, humiliation is . . . well, it's loving in its own way. Note, though, that there are different levels of intensity when it comes to humiliating factors, and some verbal abuse may trigger a traumatic feeling in the receiver. Humiliation, like other kinks, should be practiced safely and always with consent.

Voyeurism: Rita and Sean love going to sex parties, but they don't have sex with others. They're voyeurs. They love watching people get naked and have sex because it turns them on big time. It makes them super horny, and they enjoy having hot sex with each other in private after watching heated aggressive sex or an orgy. There's a difference between responsible voyeurism (such as what Rita and Sean enjoy) and voyeuristic disorder, which is when someone has urges to secretly watch people get naked or have sex without their consent. You may have heard of the term *peeping Tom*. Yeah, that's illegal and problematic. On the flip side, though, many people are responsible voyeurs, which can also be digital. Consensual digital voyeurism could be subscribers watching their favorite OnlyFans creators or cam-person doing sexual things on camera. You can also practice voyeurism in your relationship as part of a role-play. Start a video call and place your phone somewhere in the bedroom. Don't interact with your partner. Remember, you want to give the illusion of them secretly watching you. As you get naked and get ready for bed, you can throw in a little masturbation session so your partner who's "secretly watching" can get super aroused. This is a fun idea for couples who enjoy voyeuristic play without involving others. For an in-person observation, I think play/sex parties are the best places to satisfy your kinky desires.

Edging or orgasm control: "You can't cum until I say so, Michael," said Jane, his wife of eight years. Who knew orgasm control could be so stimulating? While orgasm control/denial is a part of BDSM, edging—the practice of stimulating the genitals to the point of orgasm only to stop and withhold the orgasm—has become a popular practice in the last few years. The benefit of the practice is that you can repeat it as many times as you'd like. Some people do it once, then they cum the next time; others do it more than twenty times and don't cum at all. Edging by yourself can be great for your sexual health because it helps you control your own orgasms. For men who experience premature ejaculation or are unable to orgasm, edging can be a huge benefit. It can also help women experience a more significant orgasm. Doesn't everyone want to cum?! Yes, orgasms are delicious, but some people really enjoy the act of orgasm delay or deprivation, especially when done with a partner. Just imagine—your partner manually stimulates you and your arousal is building and building until you almost orgasm, then they stop and say, "No, you can't cum until I say so!" Isn't that kinda hot? Orgasm control is a part of power play because the person with power tells the other what they can and can't do. Sex and power can be perceived very similarly. Both are inherent to human needs and desires, both can be enacted in healthy and unhealthy ways, and both exist in a Venn diagram: power is sexy, and sex is powerful. Considering that orgasms are a powerful experience, being able to induce, delay, or deny one is such a mindfuck. I think it allows for couples to feel closer together because you really need to surrender to and trust each other while engaging in orgasm control.

Food play: You read about John and Brenda at the beginning of this chapter. Their story is one way to do food play, but there are so many ways to enact this sexual fetish. The idea of food play derives from people's obsession with food and sex—literally the two most important factors of pure survival of the species. We can't evolve without food and sex, which makes food play, in a sense, very instinctual and raw. I like food play, although it's not a fetish for me. I think it's fun and exciting to involve food in some sexual practices, such as using coconut oil for ass eating or honey for nipple play. It introduces new sensory experiences to sex, particularly taste. People who have a food play fetish are aroused by the idea and act of erotic moments and practices involving food. Taking a body shot or drinking alcohol off someone's body is a practice popularized in nightlife/parties. Japanese people have their own sexy version of this called *wakame sake,* or seaweed sake. This is where a naked female partner lays down, closes her legs tight (forming a bushy triangle in her pubic area), and then has sake poured into her pelvic region, creating a "seaweed sake," while her partner devours it. Even if this is not your fetish, you can still enjoy food play. You can use honey, coconut oil, whipped cream, chocolate syrup, agave syrup, strawberries, champagne, or Popsicles in different ways with the nipples, lower back, butthole, clitoris, back of the neck, lips, penis, ass, thighs, lips, or mouth. A warning, though: I don't recommend penetration with food because it can fuck up the body's pH and cause irritation and itching in the vagina and on the penis.

Exhibitionism: I'm an exhibitionist and not ashamed of it. It's arousing for me when people watch me get fucked either lovingly or aggressively. This is one of the reasons why I enjoy sex parties—not necessarily to participate in an orgy but to have hot sex with my husband while other attendees watch. We put on exhibitions everywhere. At our old high-rise apartment, we used to have sex on the balcony because even the idea that someone *might* be watching us was a turn-on. I'm a responsible exhibitionist, so I like the idea that the people watching me have sex are enjoying it as much as I do—in a mutually consensual way. This should not be confused with exhibitionistic disorder, which is a condition where someone enjoys showing their genitals to nonconsenting strangers. Everybody I know who loves having others see them nude or watch them have sex are responsible exhibitionists in proper contexts, such as play parties, sex clubs, nude beaches, and such. How can you enjoy responsible exhibitionism for fun? For starters, you can try kissing in public or recording a video of you naked, masturbating, or having sex. You can try applying for and attending sex parties. You can also try amateur porn or online erotic work through sites like OnlyFans. (Yes, there are risks associated with all this, so proceed with caution.) Why are people into exhibitionism? There are many possible explanations. Sex is still considered a taboo activity, especially when it's not in a private space, so exhibitionism is a beautiful mix of rebellion, novelty, excitement, and acts of antisocial norms.

Cuckolding: "I just love watching my wife get absolutely railed by Smack," said Josh. Fiona responded, "It feels so empowering and hot that I get to do this, but I still feel ashamed because it's not like we can ever talk about this with anyone! They'd probably stop being friends with us." Josh and Fiona are into cuckolding, and their regular bull is Smack. Smack is a 6′3″ guy with a 9″ dick they met on a kinky dating app. Fiona's shame is not uncalled for and is sadly a valid concern. I've heard many stories of people getting shunned by their friends and family after they find out about their cuckolding practices. Cuckolding is still very much a taboo and heavily stigmatized sexual activity and way of life. What is it? It's a sexual fetish that involves watching your partner having consensual sex with someone else. The person watching is a cuck. It's traditionally practiced by heterosexual couples where the man is the cuck and his wife is fucked by a big bull (a guy with a huge cock), but it's now practiced by all kinds of people from different genders, cultures, and sexual orientations. Why is anyone into this? Well, some people are aroused by jealousy, but it can also be liberating to not be possessive of your partner and to share. It also plays into the idea that adultery is seen as sinful in most religions, so the antireligious nature of cuckolding can be a turn-on for many. It's also not a new practice; it's just talked about more openly now. In his book *Insatiable Wives*[39], Dr. David Ley claims that cuckolding can be dated back to the thirteenth century. There are rules and proper ways to engage in this activity, so make sure you research it thoroughly and don't do it haphazardly. Of course, a lot of open and honest communication and trust is involved in cuckolding relationships. If you're into this practice or this type of relationship, there's nothing wrong with you. It can be hard to find a partner who understands and wants to participate in this lifestyle, but Venus Cuckoldress, an expert and enthusiast, has started a matchmaking service for cucks called Venus Connections. Try it out, y'all.

Hotpast: "My ex's cock was so much bigger than yours. One time he fucked me in the bathroom at a rooftop bar, and he made me squirt everywhere. I came so hard for him." This is what I used to say to one of my exes (let's use a fake name), Peter. Peter had a huge hotpast kink. He loved it when I talked about my exes and my past sexual experiences. He loved it so much that sometimes he'd record me talking about having sex with an ex and then listen to it while masturbating at home. Hotpast is a bit like humiliation but not exactly the same. It's all verbal communication—talking about the past. It involves talking about sex with your ex, your ex's genitals, one of your past hookups or one-night stands, one of your past orgasm experiences, and so on. Is it common? Not especially, but it's not unusual. The subreddit r/hotpast has more than 106,000 (primarily male) members. Are women into

---

39. Carolee A. Kallmann, "A Review of 'Insatiable Wives: Women Who Stray and the Men Who Love Them,'" *Journal of Sex & Marital Therapy* 36, no. 5 (September 2010): 449–451, https://doi.org/10.1080/0092623x.2010.512228.

this kink? They are, but it's not as common. Why are people into it? Well, psychologist Dr. David Ley called it an eroticization of fear where people turn something they're afraid of into something empowering in an effort to reclaim themselves through that fear. Another reason why some people find it enjoyable is retrospective jealousy: jealousy of someone's past sexual experiences. Jealousy is a powerful emotion, and if someone can turn that into sexual arousal, it's safe to say it can be sexually powerful. It's also safer than invoking jealousy by thinking your partner is cheating on you, which can cause paranoia since that focuses on the present. There are a few ways people engage in a hotpast kink. It could just be hearing a story about a past sexual encounter, or they could add a humiliation layer by making comparisons. In a way, it's kind of like cuckolding but without sex with someone else. In 2018, a research paper[40] was published in the Archives of Sexual Behaviors claiming that fulfilling a fantasy of partner-sharing can be positive and healthy for couples. You may be into this kink or can't imagine ever doing it, but as long as it's fun for the couple, then who are we to judge? I treated Peter respectfully, like I did with other lovers. His kink didn't make me evaluate him poorly in any way. He was a fun and cool guy, and it was a great relationship while it lasted. (It didn't end because of his kink, by the way.)

BDSM: A lot of people still judge it as a taboo lifestyle, but BDSM is way more commonly practiced than you might think. Your dentist, farmer, bus driver, lawyer, and barista could be going to the same BDSM club. If you google BDSM, you'll get more than 30 million results. Though it's still stigmatized, BDSM relationships and the lifestyle are increasingly popular. BDSM is a general term for people who engage in various practices for pleasure, connection, and sexual gratification that are considered a mix of nontraditional sexual behaviors and power play.

---

40. Justin J. Lehmiller, David Ley, and Dan Savage, "The Psychology of Gay Men's Cuckolding Fantasies," *Archives of Sexual Behavior* 47, no. 4 (May 2018): 999–1013, https://pubmed.ncbi.nlm.nih.gov/29285655/.

Bondage (B) is an erotic practice that involves restraining and tying up one's sexual partner. Although bondage is more popular in Western countries such as the United States and Germany, Japan has its own bondage practice called *Shibari* that started in the 1400s. Originally, it was to bind captives of war, but it evolved into a mindful bondage practice within the sexual realm. In bondage, the person who is tying up is called a *rigger*, and the person who enjoys being tied up is called a *rope bunny*. Traditionally, men have tied up women, but that dynamic has changed over time and nowadays, just about anyone can be tied up. Bondage is usually practiced within the realm of a BDSM relationship but not always. Millions of couples have tried using handcuffs in bed, which is a light form of bondage and an interesting way to play with restraint, even if you don't practice other facets of BDSM. Let me be clear: Bondage can be dangerous. If you're going to practice it, you need to establish some rules, such as never leaving the rope bunny tied up alone in case something happens, never tying the restraints so hard that the rope bunny starts bleeding (unless that's part of the kink), and never using illegitimate ropes (ropes not made specifically for bondage and Shibari).

Discipline/Dominance (D) is the practice of training the submissive partner (sub) to obey the rules. When the sub breaks the rules, they receive punishment for their disobedience in various forms of physical, mental, or emotional punishment. Disciplining a sub can include, but is not limited to, spanking, caning, whipping, gagging, verbally attacking, ignoring, or humiliating them. Discipline is a big part of the Dom and Sub (D/s) or master and slave relationship. The dom is a dom because they tell the sub what to do, and the sub must yield and obey, which makes it a functionable BDSM relationship. Without discipline, it's not power play; safe words are vital. Even though the kink is about inflicting pain to punish the sub erotically, it still needs to be within an acceptable realm of pain for the sub. Therefore, if the sub yells out the safe word, the punishment must be stopped. Newbies, of course, can practice BDSM in a less intense way with "funishments" (fun + punishments): sexy spanking and other light activities.

Sadism (S) is the tendency to derive sexual pleasure from inflicting physical, mental, and emotional pain on a sexual partner. Flogging a partner, attacking them verbally, or using nipple clamps are some of the ways a sadist can inflict pain for sexual gratification. By contrast, masochism (M) is the tendency to derive sexual pleasure from receiving physical, mental, or emotional pain from a sexual partner. A masochist may enjoy getting flogged, slapped, called derogatory names, ball-gagged, and sensory deprived. S&M is practiced as a duo. A sadist is nothing without their masochist, and vice versa. The term *sadism* derives from the name of French author/aristocrat Marquis de Sade who wrote books that involved sadistic sexual activities like sexual violence and coercion. *The 120 Days of Sodom* is the story of four French libertines who lock themselves and multiple victims in a mansion for four months and subject the victims to emotional and sexual tortures. The book was and is extremely controversial, often showing up on banned book lists. The term *masochism* comes from the name of Austrian author Leopold von Sacher-Masoch who wrote about the sexual satisfaction he gained from being whipped, dominated, and humiliated.

BDSM can be practiced in varying degrees but should always be done with consent. Beginners may enjoy light BDSM where they use handcuffs at home for bondage, an eye mask for sensory deprivation, and some light spanking. People who enjoy this lifestyle often choose to intensify their experiences in many different ways. If this sexual practice and lifestyle tickles your interest, I encourage you to spend time researching how you want to practice it and how much you want to be involved. There are BDSM classes, sex clubs, and events in most big cities so you can find others in this community to learn from and bond with. Community is such a big part of BDSM because it's still a misunderstood practice, but within the community you can feel accepted and appreciated.

Domination and submission: D/s is a part of BDSM. Many practitioners will tell you that D/s is more about exchanging power and navigating power dynamics than it is about sex. The dom is the leader in the relationship or sexual encounter, and the sub is the follower. Some people live 24/7 dom-and-sub lives while others enact it only during sexual encounters or via role-play. The whole D/s subculture is extensive. There are rules and norms, tight communities, and celebrations through parties and parades. There are countless blogs, books, and research studies on this lifestyle, so I highly recommend you read up on this topic as much as you can if you're interested.

Let's get some myths out of the way regarding BDSM and D/s. Are BDSM practitioners mentally ill? No. Do all of them have a history of sexual trauma? No. Are they all violent in real life? No. Sure, there are some people that may fit that description, but there are also priests and CEOs who are mentally ill, have sexual traumas, and are violent—but they're rarely subjected to the same judgments that BDSM practitioners are. Although people tend to think of men as doms and women as subs, there are many amateur and professional dominatrixes of all genders. I had the pleasure of interviewing three—Damiana Chi, PhD, Colette Pervette, and Eva Oh—and learned so much about this lifestyle. Curious? Feel free to listen to their episodes of *Luvbites by Dr. Tara* to learn more.

There are also many categories of D/s. Financial domination (findom) has been in the spotlight recently due to the prominence of the internet and social media. This is the practice where the sub gives money and gifts to the dom. In findom, the sub doesn't expect any sexual interaction from the dom. They just get off on the idea of giving them money and gifts. There's also master/servant relationships, where the service sub serves the master in other, nonsexual contexts of life (e.g., making their bed, cooking for them, cleaning their space, or helping them in other ways). Another D/s relationship that is becoming more popular is puppy play. This is where the dom is the owner and the sub is a puppy. The "puppy" can be brushed, bathed, and taken out for a walk on a leash. People enjoy these unique types of relationships for various reasons, including sexual pleasure, relaxation, and escapism—even therapeutic reasons. I believe all types of sexual relationships can be amazing as long as they're legal, consensual, and pleasurable.

AFTERCARE

Aftercare is an extremely important aspect of kinks and fetishes. Have you ever heard of people saying they feel *used* after sex? This often happens when there isn't any proper aftercare: the practice of physically, emotionally, or mentally tending to your partner after sex. It's particularly important after kinky sex because there could be physical pain that needs tending to or emotional and mental bruises that need more TLC, but I think it should be practiced by everybody. Aftercare practices can include physical aftercare (e.g., massaging your partner or cleaning their body) and emotional and mental aftercare (e.g., talking about the sex session as a recap, giving compliments, cuddling, kissing, caressing). Ask your partner how they like to be cared for after sex. Interestingly, some people just enjoy some alone time right after sex because they want the space to calm down. It's always good to ask their preferences and share yours.

COMMUNICATING YOUR KINK

"I want to see you get fucked by someone else," Dave said during sex with Janice. Janice responded rather abruptly, "Whoa, whoa! What the fuck, Dave? Get off me. What do you mean?"

That's a real (bad) example from one of my clients and a reminder that you should never share your kink haphazardly. It needs to be well thought out and communicated clearly in the right context. In this example, Janice was concerned after Dave shared his cuckolding fantasy that he wanted to fulfill in real life. After a lot of damage control, rebuilding trust, and talking through it, Janice started to understand Dave's cuckolding desires. They ended up trying it digitally in a controlled environment: Janice had cybersex with someone they met online while Dave watched and masturbated.

Here are my tips for communicating your desires for unconventional sex: ADORE.

1. **Ask Questions: Ask your partner what they currently know about the kink. You can gauge their perception and knowledge of it, which can help you navigate the conversation.**

2. **Discuss: It should always be a discussion—not a demand or request. People can get defensive if they feel like they're being asked to try kinky sex because they may feel like they don't have any control over it. After asking questions, share your interests and passion in the kink. Make it a discussion session.**

3. **(Maintain) an Open Mind: This is key when it comes to talking about kinks and fetishes. Don't yuck other people's yum. There's no kink shaming or vanilla shaming.**

4. **Revisit Later: You don't have to get to the bottom of things in the first discussion. Be patient and have the initial conversation knowing you'll revisit the topic later (potentially many times before it is enacted).**

5. **(Have) Empathy: This is needed both ways. The kinkster and their partner need to engage in serious conversations about nontraditional sexual behaviors with empathy. Try to understand your partner and put yourself in their shoes. Ultimately, everyone wants to be loved and desired, so be gentle and empathetic as you talk about kinks and fetishes.**

Here's what this can look like:

"Hey babe, have you ever heard of cuckolding? I listened to a podcast about it yesterday. It's interesting." If they've never heard of it, you can proceed with, "I'll send you a link to the podcast. I'd love for you to listen to it and let me know what you think." If they've heard about it before, you can continue talking about the kink. "What do you think of it?" "How do you feel about it?" "I have a feeling I might be into it. When they explained how it works, I just thought . . . that's hot. It's something I might want to explore in the future."

As a receiver, it's important to respond with empathy and not immediately react with something like, "Ugh, that's gross" or "I don't know why anyone would be into that." Instead, focus on an empathetic and open-minded response like, "Wow, thanks for sharing with me. This is a lot, and I want to process it and look into it more, but I'm open to talking through another day, if that's OK."

Of course, this is just one example, but you get the idea. The key thing is that when you share your kinks, you want to make it a discussion, not a demand or request, and as a receiver, you always want to withhold judgment and try to understand your partner, even if it's something you won't want to do. Lead these sensitive conversations with love and compassion.

A SHAMELESS WORLD

Wouldn't it be nice if we lived in a shameless world? Like, it's cool if you have kinks and fetishes, and it's cool if you don't. The first time I realized that I was nontraditional—because I wanted to explore sex parties with my partner—I felt so much shame. It felt shameful to want anything else but a traditional relationship and marriage. It felt shameful as a woman to have the desire to explore group sex. It felt shameful to be OK with my partner enjoying pleasure with others. But all that changed when I started to accept myself for who I am. I started going to therapy and embarked on a personal development journey. Now, I explore unapologetically with my loving husband, and it's been amazing. In my ideal world, I'd love for people to curiously explore at their own pace and decide for themselves what's pleasurable and fun for them. No kink or vanilla shaming allowed. Let the people do what they desire and live their best lives!

Chapter 6

Let's Talk About Sex, Baby: Macro Sexual Communication

To effectively communicate, we must realize that we are all different in the way we perceive the world and use this understanding as a guide to our communication with others.

—Tony Robbins

"Hey babe, on a scale of one to ten, how would you rate your sex life last month?" I suggested Amy ask her husband, Jason, this question.

"Are you serious? I can't ask that. He's going to think there's something wrong with our sex life or I'm not happy," Amy worried. "Anything I bring up is going to make him feel defensive."

"Well, be honest with me . . . are you happy?" I said lovingly but with a note of sass. "For the last thirty minutes, you've been telling me that your sex life is as dull as a hundred-year-old knife. I think it's time for a proper sexy check-in."

"I guess you're right," Amy admitted. "Ugh, I really don't want to do it."

That's the thing; I believe most people, like Amy, know it's important to talk about sexual preferences, concerns, desires, and boundaries with their partner, but they're afraid to bring it up and don't really know how to start. The simple truth is that talking about sex can feel really hard when you've never done it before. Why? Because sex is still taboo in our society, and talking about it can sometimes feel like it's harder than doing it. However, like most skill-based activities, you will get better and more comfortable with it every time you do it. Amy started talking about her sexual concerns in our first session, brought her husband to our fourth session, and then began talking about sex regularly. It works when you start trying.

Easier said than done, right? Trust me, I know exactly how you feel. It took me years to feel comfortable communicating my own sexual needs and desires.

For me, talking about sex and advocating for my sexual desires is a way to gain more self-respect and build my confidence. The myth that you have to become confident before you have the courage to talk about and advocate for your sexual well-being is, frankly, BS. You don't need to wait. You don't need to be 100 percent confident. Like Amy, you can be 60 percent confident and good to go. This is similar to the narrative people believe about being in a healthy relationship: "Oh, I need to fix myself first. I need to be whole first before I'm worthy to date anyone." Again, that's BS. When you're in the right relationship, you grow together. No one is perfect, and you don't need to wait until you're "perfect" to deserve love, pleasure, and sexual satisfaction. You're fine as long as you continuously improve and have a growth mindset.

In my current marriage with Brent, we talk about sex regularly, doing sexy check-ins, asking about desires and reservations, and talking about our sex party experiences. With him, it's much easier now than it was when we started dating. At the beginning, he wasn't a great communicator, but he trusted me to initiate those conversations and continuously improved his communication skills because of his growth mindset. At first, it was awkward for him to share his desires and needs, but over time, he learned that I wouldn't judge him for what he was telling me. When you have a shared belief and trust, it's a much easier task.

I want to highlight two caveats here. First, I'm the person who initiates most of our sex conversations—and that's OK. I hear from a lot of people who they wish their partners would bring up the topic of sex so they can have an open conversation. I always ask, "Why not you? Why can't it be you who brings up the conversation?" You need to clarify expectations so the two of you can create a sexual communication protocol that works. Start the first conversation, then mention that you want them to initiate the next conversation. Make it a monthly thing—a normal, regular, healthy conversation between the two of you (or include a coach or therapist). The second caveat is that there must be a judgment-free zone. I've created a sense of open-mindedness in my relationship where my partner feels he can share anything, and we can always talk it out—whether I agree with the topic under discussion or not. This is what I call a *curiosity-led relationship,* meaning both partners approach every conversation with a curious mind and want to understand each other and make things work. Curious people are generally less judgmental and defensive and more interested in the why and how. For example, in a relationship not guided by curiosity, one partner may think, "Ugh, I hate that my boyfriend acts submissive in bed. That's so weird. It's way hotter when men are dominant." By contrast, in a curiosity-led relationship, that person may think, "Why does my partner love being submissive in bed? How can we make it work together since we both enjoy being submissive?"

There's a large body of research[41] that suggests sexual communication is vital to long-term sexual satisfaction, and how satisfied you are with your sex life contributes greatly to your overall relationship satisfaction (with the exception of asexual people). The two go together like chocolate and peanut butter, champagne and caviar, foreplay and orgasms. An unfulfilling sex life can sneak up on you and before you know it, you're

41. Allen B. Mallory, "Dimensions of Couples' Sexual Communication, Relationship Satisfaction, and Sexual Satisfaction: A Meta-Analysis," *Journal of Family Psychology* 36, no. 3 (April 2022): 358–371, https://doi.org/10.1037/fam0000946; Byers, "Relationship Satisfaction and Sexual Satisfaction," 113–118.

crying in the bathroom because you haven't had an orgasm in a long time or you're flirtatiously texting your ex because you don't feel desired by your current partner. However, many of the potential consequences can be prevented with macro sexual communication: conversations about your sex life as an individual and together as a couple.

In this chapter, I will explain different types of sex conversations and show you how to have those conversations with your date/partner/spouse, based on proven methods from research, my professional experience as a coach, and my personal experience going from an anxious sexual communicator to an unashamed and outspoken sexpert. I've learned to talk about sex confidently and unapologetically, and you can too! I promise.

WHY IS IT HARD FOR PEOPLE TO TALK ABOUT SEX?

Sex is a sensitive topic for several reasons, but most people find it difficult to talk about because of cultural norms and a lack of education. Talking about sex, sexual pleasure, or sex issues in most cultures—especially among women—is taboo. The narrative is that sex is just something you naturally do with your committed partner, and that's it. We all know that communication is key to a happy relationship, yet it's still hard to shake off hundreds of years of sexual communication norms. In addition, most people don't ever receive comprehensive sex education that teaches how to start these conversations and what to talk about. Without proper education and information, sexual communication can be intimidating and anxiety-inducing.

The Uncertainty Reduction Theory[42] suggests people often experience uncertainty in interpersonal interactions and relationships, which creates cognitive stress and anxiety. That's why they use communication

---

42. Leanne K. Knobloch, "Uncertainty Reduction Theory," *International Encyclopedia of Interpersonal Communication,* December 2015, 1–9, https://doi.org/10.1002/9781118540190.wbeic144.

to gain more information, gain a better understanding of the person and situation, and reduce uncertainty. People tend like each other more when there's less uncertainty. This is why communicating about sex can make your sex life so much more orgasmic. Talking about your preferences, likes, and dislikes helps your partner reduce uncertainty and become more "fluent" in having sex with you. Research[43] also shows that most people wish their partners would tell them directly what gives them pleasure rather than just let them guess. I think it's time we all quit the guessing game so we can play and make sure everyone's happy.

Sexual communication anxiety is also very real. I did a poll on my Instagram and wasn't surprised to see that 53 percent of people reported having sexual communication anxiety: that nervous feeling you have when talking about or anticipating a conversation about sex. I've personally and professionally observed people feeling anxious about sexual communication on all kinds of issues. My sister said talking to her partner about sex toys in their bedroom makes her nervous. A friend told me she's anxious to bring up the topic of her boyfriend's penis size (it's smaller than what she's used to). A client said they are afraid to bring up the topic of opening up the relationship and sexually exploring with other people together. These are different issues but result in similar experiences.

Communication just takes practice to feel more comfortable. It is truly a skill. The more you do it, thc morc you become confident and fluent at it, but the effectiveness of sexual communication also has relationship prerequisites. First, you need trust. If you don't trust your partner, then there's no way you're going to have the capacity to open up and share such vulnerable thoughts and feelings. When you trust your partner, you trust that they love you, won't judge you, and want the best for you. Therefore, trust allows you to openly communicate your sexual desires, needs, and

---

43. Elaine Hatfield and Richard L. Rapson, *Love, Sex, and Intimacy: Their Psychology, Biology, and History* (HarperCollins College Publishers, 1996).

concerns. Without trust, it's difficult to share something so raw and personal, so building strong trust in a relationship is vital. And how do we build strong trust? Well, a lot of it comes from consistency and positive interactions. You want to do the things you say you'll do; following through creates a sense of trust. Put in the effort to make most of your interactions positive. How you deal with arguments and conflict can be constructive, rather than through personal attacks or by giving the cold shoulder.

Societal pressure is also a big part of it. So many of us were taught that sex isn't something you talk about. If you mentioned it as a teenager, I bet you immediately got shut down by your parents and teachers as if it were something wrong. I think it's sad that something so natural and beautiful became so taboo and secretive. Far too many people grow up without positive role models of healthy sexual communication. It just hasn't been a part of our societal norm. This was clearly illustrated during a conversation I had with a guy at a dinner party.

He said, "If you're talking about sex, you ain't having any!" He challenged me with this uninformed opinion after I told him what I do for work, but his reaction is likely because that's what he's heard and been told all his life.

"Well, it's not too late to change your mind and start having conversations about sex so your second wife doesn't leave you," I responded jokingly—but he started to look very serious.

"How did you know I just got a divorce?" he asked curiously. He's been my client now for more than six months, and I'm proud to say he's becoming a great communicator. So yeah, people can change—even skeptics.

We all make assumptions. "If he likes me enough, he'll go down on me without me telling him." "I think my wife likes when I bite her nipples." "If she wanted me to wear a condom, she would have said something." "If my partner didn't like getting spanked, he would have told me." "If my blowjobs are good, he should moan louder." "I think my boyfriend is cheating on me. He's not having sex with me so he must be having sex with someone else." "I assume my wife is asexual because she hasn't initiated sex with me for over a year." "My boyfriend is so insecure, he doesn't even want to use sex toys." "I'm sure my girlfriend will think I'm a fucking loser if I tell her that I'm into being a submissive."

Ahh! I wish more people knew that communication is a superpower and their assumptions are often wrong. Assumptions can create resentment, negative feelings toward your partner, and low self-esteem. When you assume that things are worse than they actually are, you're creating hell for yourself without really learning the other person's truths. Maybe it's a completely different story than the one you've been telling yourself. Even I've fallen for the assumption game. I'm guilty of thinking my boyfriend was cheating on me because he wasn't having sex with me. In truth, though, his experience was, "I'm so ashamed that I haven't had any sex drive lately, and I'm afraid she'll think I'm not masculine enough." These assumptions caused us a lot of undue emotional distress. Open communication is the best way to combat unnecessary emotional pain caused by assumptions and misunderstandings.

BENEFITS OF SEXUAL COMMUNICATION

The benefits of sexual communication are immense, so a few paragraphs won't do it justice, but I'll try. In the research I presented at my TEDx talk[44], I surveyed five thousand people in long-term relationships to figure out what variables were the most important factors contributing to high sexual satisfaction. The data strongly relayed that sexual communication is one of the strongest predictors of long-term sexual satisfac-

44. Tara Suwinyattichaipoirn, "Become Sexually Powerful," TEDx CSUF, Fullerton, CA, December 2, 2021, 11 min., 9 sec., https://www.youtube.com/watch?v=u-tkbBnmfbw.

tion. Without proper communication about the kind of sex life that you desire, it's unlikely that you are having satisfying sex after the so-called honeymoon phase has faded away. People tend to experience this initial phase of a relationship through rose-tinted glasses and see everything as rainbows and butterflies. I love that new-love energy; it's exciting and so much fun. As you continue to learn more about and spend time with each other, though, the relationship develops. That initial sense of excitement shifts to a different sense of closeness, trust, and a stronger bond. This is incredible, but the truth is that the sex also changes. A new sense of sexual intimacy needs to be established after the honeymoon phase, and that's only possible if both partners are regularly talking about their sexual needs, desires, and boundaries.

Another study[45] found sexual communication is correlated with increased orgasm frequency. More orgasms? Who doesn't like that? It's music to my ears. If being more satisfied with your sex life and having more orgasms doesn't convince you to start talking about sex, I don't know what else will. The researchers found that women who experience more orgasms report higher levels of relationship satisfaction. I can attest to this finding, not because I'm shallow and just want to cum but because I know for a fact that female orgasms are often (though not always) correlated with how other aspects of the relationship are going. If there's trust, love, open communication, and positivity—and if both partners are putting in the effort to maintain the relationship—then women are more able to experience pleasure in bed. This may all sound fairly obvious, but there's a flipside: People who don't communicate about sex often report higher levels of sexual dissatisfaction[46]. This resonates so much in my practice.

---

45. Adam C. Jones et al., "The Role of Sexual Communication in Couples' Sexual Outcomes: A Dyadic Path Analysis," *Journal of Marital and Family Therapy* 44, no. 4 (October 2017): 606–623, https://doi.org/10.1111/jmft.12282.
46. Jennifer L. Montesi et al., "On the Relationship Among Social Anxiety, Intimacy, Sexual Communication, and Sexual Satisfaction in Young Couples," *Archives of Sexual Behavior* 42, no. 1 (April 2012): 81–91, https://doi.org/10.1007/s10508-012-9929-3.

The common denominator among clients who are extremely frustrated with their current sex lives is a lack of communication about sex.

Sexual self-esteem is also significantly linked to sexual communication. It's a reciprocal relationship. When you talk about sex more often, you feel more confident and self-assured, which contributes to a higher level of self-esteem because you know you can advocate for your own sexual well-being. When you have high sexual self-esteem[47], you will express yourself in a more confident way and be more likely to discuss your sexual needs with your partner. Having high sexual self-esteem is important because that's when you know you're worthy of pleasure, connection, and being treated respectfully (or consensually disrespectfully if that's the way you roll). Sexual self-esteem and sexual confidence are powerful, linked factors in a healthy sex life. In addition, a stronger bond[48] and sense of happiness about the relationship are definite benefits of talking about sex. When you overcome a hard situation together, it makes your connection stronger, affirms your bond, and brings more joy to the relationship.

WHAT EXACTLY IS SEXUAL COMMUNICATION?

People always look perplexed when I tell them I teach sexual communication at a university. Some common responses I've received over the years are, "What does that even mean?" "Whoa, they didn't have that kind of class when I went to college!" and "I don't think I need it but tell me what it's about." I know y'all are ready to learn, so let's get to it.

---

47. M. K. Oattes and A. Offman, "Global Self-Esteem and Sexual Self-Esteem as Predictors of Sexual Communication in Intimate Relationships," *Canadian Journal of Human Sexuality* no. 3 (January 2007): 89–100.
48. Sheila MacNeil and E. Sandra Byers, "Dyadic Assessment of Sexual Self-Disclosure and Sexual Satisfaction in Heterosexual Dating Couples," *Journal of Social and Personal Relationships* 22, no. 2 (April 2005): 169–181, https://doi.org/10.1177/0265407505050942.

Sexual communication consists of macro and micro communication (the latter is detailed in the next chapter). Macro sexual communication consists of conversations about your sex life, sexual preferences, desires, needs, interests, boundaries, and so on. It's the conversations you have to obtain, maintain, and enhance a healthy sex life for yourself and your partner. Whether you just started dating, have been in a relationship for a while, or have been together with a committed partner for a long time, it's never too late to start having these conversations.

How do you start? Here are five ways to start talking about sex:

Initiate an in-person disclosure: Directly tell your partner that you want to start talking about each other's sexual preferences and interests. Initiate the conversation in a nonsexual setting, such as over coffee, during lunch or dinner, or while on a hike. This makes it easier because you're probably already in a conversational mode in those contexts. For new partners, you can say, "I know we just started dating, but I really like you and want us to be on the same page sexually. Would you be open to talking about sex? / Can we talk about our sexual preferences? / Are you down to talk about what we like and dislike in bed?" Alternatively, you could say, "We've not yet talked about sex, and it's OK, but I want us to be honest about what we like and dislike in bed, and I think now is a good time to start. What do you think?" If you've been together for a long time, try saying, "I know we've been together for a while, but we've never actually talked about sex. I'm thankful we've had great sex, so I'm excited for us to dive deeper into our sexual interests and create an even stronger sexual connection. What do you think?" Alternatively, you could say, "I recently read a book about how sexual communication is very important in long-term relationships and enhances sexual connection. I know we've never talked about sex before, but I'd love to start having conversations about our sex life together. Would you be open to it?"

Initiate an e-disclosure: Text your partner that you want to start talking about each other's sexual preferences and interests. This is much more common for people in new relationships, but if you're in a long-term relationship and are more comfortable initiating a conversation with your partner via text, this could be the right strategy for you. This only works if texting is your normal method of communication. Don't text if it's unusual for you. For new relationships, you can text, "I know we've just started seeing each other, but I really like you and want us to be on the same page sexually. Are you open to talking about sexual preferences and interests?" For long-term couples, text, "I just finished a book about sexual well-being, and the author talks about how vital sexual communication is for long-term partners to maintain a healthy sex life. I'd love for us to talk about it when you get home! What do you think?"

Share credible social media posts and online articles: Send your partner links to articles or social media posts from credible sources as cues that you want to discuss the topic. For example, if you want to start talking about trying anal sex, you can share a relevant article from *Healthline* or *WebMD* with the message "Can we talk about this tomorrow? ;-)" Maybe you want to talk about BDSM, so you can share a social media post from a credible source (e.g., credentialed content creators or legit organizations) with the message "Thoughts on this topic? :)"

Gift a book: Books are great to help people feel more comfortable about the topic of sex. Be careful about which book you choose, though, and how you gift it. I once saw a husband give his wife a book about polyamory without any explanation, and it went terribly. (They came in for coaching after that happened to mitigate further conflict.) The best books for sexual communication newbies are more neutral titles, such as this book, *Come as You Are* by Emily Nagoski, *She Comes First* by Ian Kerner, *Better Sex Through Mindfulness* by Lori Brotto, and *Smart Sex* by Emily Morse. See the resource library at the end of this book for more recommended reading materials. When gifting a book, you need to attach a message, such as "I heard it's a great read!" or "It's an awesome read! Let me know what you think." You can even read the book together with your partner(s).

Try a sex and relationship app: Are you tech savvy? There are many mobile apps out there that can facilitate initial conversations about sex without the awkwardness. For example, Couply is a great relationship app that can help you communicate your sexual preferences, kinks, and desires. If you experience a lot of sexual communication anxiety, it's not a bad idea to begin by playing a game on an app together. It's low risk and less threatening than initiating a direct conversation.

DOS AND DON'TS OF MACRO SEXUAL COMMUNICATION

Dos	Don'ts
• Use a soft tone of voice. • Make meaningful eye contact. • Try to be empathetic and understand your partner's point of view. • Listen attentively; don't just listen to respond. • Meditate and visualize a successful conversation before having it.	• Don't use a negative tone of voice (e.g., sarcastic, nagging, threatening). • Don't interrupt your partner mid-thought. • Don't avoid eye contact. • Don't be defensive. • Don't listen to respond without trying to understand.

THIRTY SEX QUESTIONS TO ASK YOUR PARTNER

Of course, there are plenty more questions you can ask each other, but if you break through that first barrier and get through these fifty questions, you'll be able to talk about anything sex related for all the years to come without anxiety and shame.

1. **When do you think people/couples should talk about sex?**

2. **How do you feel about sexual communication/having conversations about sex?**

3. **What are your sexual turn-ons (e.g., nipple play)?**

4. **How do you like me to initiate sex? Do you prefer verbal or nonverbal communication?**

5. **How often do you wish to have sex in a week or a month?**
6. **How do you like your erogenous zones stimulated?**
7. **How important is sex in long-term relationships?**
8. **How would you describe amazing sex?**
9. **What are some things I do during sex that need some adjustment?**
10. **What is one of your sexual fantasies?**
11. **How do you feel about exploring kinky sex?**
12. **What's your view on watching porn?**
13. **Would you ever explore BDSM?**
14. **How often do you think couples should try a new sexual thing?**
15. **Apart from penetration, what other sexual activities do you really enjoy?**
16. **What is something you want to sexually explore in the near future?**
17. **How do you feel about scheduling sex?**
18. **What activities help you "get in the mood"?**
19. **What do you think about dirty talk?**
20. **How do you feel about sexting?**
21. **What do you know about tantric sex? Do you want to learn more about it?**
22. **Do you prefer dominating or being submissive—or both—in bed?**
23. **Is there something sexually unconventional that you're curious about? What is it?**
24. **What is your favorite time of day to have sex?**

25. What's one of your favorite sexual memories of us?

26. What do you think about masturbation?

27. What do you think about sex toys?

28. How would you describe great oral sex?

29. What's your view on sex parties and sex clubs?

30. How do you feel our sex life will evolve as we get older?

For more questions, you can subscribe to my newsletter at Luvbites.co. I send a new question every week for you to talk about with your partner!

ARE YOU DATING A BAD COMMUNICATOR?

BAD stands for *blaming, assumptive, and dismissive.* If your answer to the above question is *yes,* you may need couple's counseling to restructure your communication expectations and respect within the relationship—or you may need to leave the relationship if it's really *bad* because these are signs of unhealthy communication patterns that can cause a lot of anxiety, negative emotions, and poor mental health. A BAD communicator likes to blame their partner for external circumstances, especially when it comes to sex, without acknowledging their role in it. For instance, a client's husband blamed her for all the animosity he had toward her because they hadn't had sex in six months. Instead of having a constructive conversation about what a desirable sex life looks like for the both of them, he resorted to blaming her for everything.

An assumptive communicator likes to assume everything before collecting the right information. For example, a friend freaked out on her boyfriend, saying he didn't desire her anymore because he didn't ejaculate when they had sex. She thought he couldn't cum because he didn't find her sexy or attractive. In fact, he was under an incredible amount of stress because he got laid off from work and didn't have the courage to tell her yet. With that on his mind, he couldn't cum. Assumptive communicators cause more disruption than understanding in a relationship, and their behavior usually stems from their own personal insecurities.

A dismissive communicator is probably the worst of the three. They do not communicate at all, dismiss their partner's concerns, and often gaslight their partner and their experiences. One client came to a session to fix his relationship because his wife continuously dismissed his concerns about their lack of passion and gave zero effort in the sexual intimacy department. She refused to attend any of our sessions for months and told him that he was being overly dramatic about their situation. He finally came to a decision that theirs was not the kind of relationship he wanted to be in for the long run, so he filed for a divorce. It's unfortunate that their marriage had to end; as a coach, I hate seeing people going through divorce. However, sometimes divorce is the best gift because it frees both partners from a relationship that doesn't fit. Just be sure that next time around, you have a conversation about sex *before* you get married.

PROACTIVE SEXUAL COMMUNICATION: "SEXY CHECK-INS"

Talking about sex is like maintaining a car; you have to do it regularly so it doesn't break down or even explode in the middle of the freeway. It's dangerous to wait until the shit hits the fan, and, honestly, that's not mentally good for anybody. I'm therefore encouraging you to start talking about sex proactively by doing regular sexy check-ins. Maintain that beautiful car you have so it rides smoothly for a long, long time. As a society, we need to move beyond thinking that talking about sex isn't "sexy." Having this attitude ends up being a barrier between you and good sex. Say *no* to excuses and start scheduling those sexy check-ins!

- **Weekly check-in**
    - **How was our sex life this week?**
- **Monthly check-in**
    - **How would you rate our sex life this month (1–10)? Why?**
    - **What was great about it?**
    - **How can we improve that together by at least one point?**
- **Annual check-in**
    - **How was our sex life this year overall?**
    - **What's a positive memory you have of our sex life?**
    - **What's something we can improve on both individually and together?**
    - **What do we want to explore next year?**
    - **How can we start exploring that?**

SEX AS AN ACT OF COMMUNICATION

Whether you're having sex, not having sex, having amazing sex, having mediocre sex, having daytime sex, having nighttime sex, having vanilla sex, having kinky sex, having sex with each other, having a threesome—whatever it is—you're communicating something through your engagement (or lack thereof) in sexual acts. Sex sends a message, and specific sex acts communicate deep meaning (e.g., spending time pleasuring your partner, making deep eye contact, cumming together). I encourage you to always put in the effort when you have sex with your partner. Whether it's sexy foreplay, oral sex, naked cuddling, sexual meditation, or penetration, stay present and focus on your partner and the sensations in your body. When you have great sex and create a solid sexual connection with your partner, you're sending a message to each other about commitment, care, and closeness. Pay attention. No Mediocre Sex!

COMMUNICATION AFTERCARE

It's important to make sure that you and your partner both feel good about the sex-related conversations you have. Macro sexual communication can feel like a huge task because it is a lot of information to process and there are many barriers to overcome. With that in mind, be empathetic and always check in with each other. Make sure the conversation went well and both of you feel heard, respected, and understood. After all, those are basic requirements for a happy relationship.

Chapter 7

Talk Dirty to Me: Micro Sexual Communication

Just because you're my princess doesn't mean I won't fuck you like a slut.

—Ella Dominguez, *Continental Life*

Verbalizing your pleasure and discomfort during sex can feel hella awkward if you've never tried it before, but (like anal) it definitely gets easier the more you do it. Jessica was a self-proclaimed terrible communicator, to the detriment of all her past relationships. She didn't know how to express herself during sex, so she was always a silent lover and, in her own words, "weird and robotic." Until recently, she had been casually hooking up with strangers and colleagues, which was easy because she didn't have to try to improve her communication skills with casual fucks and one-night stands. However, all that changed once she started dating Tim. She fell in love with him, and that propelled her to improve her communication in bed. Although they've been dating for six months and their sex life is "pretty good," she still had inhibitions about expressing herself during sex, which led her to decide that she wanted to change. That's when she came to my coaching practice.

"How do I just let go and not give a fuck?" she asked.

After a few sessions of unpacking, we learned that Jessica's inhibitions stemmed from her first sexual encounter with her high school boyfriend. At that point, she had seen porn and wanted to say something dirty in bed, so she moaned, "Oh yeah, daddy!"

He stopped and said, "Jess, that's so fucking weird. I don't like it." Even though it seems like a small incident, it stuck with her. Ever since, she has limited her expressions in bed—both verbal and nonverbal—because she didn't want her sexual partner to freak out. During our sessions, she learned more about what healthy sexual communication is and how her high school boyfriend's response had nothing to do with her, which helped her understand that dirty talk is not a bad thing. In fact, it's a great thing!

We also practiced positive affirmation journaling, sexual meditation, and moaning exercises together. After a few months, Jessica became more comfortable communicating during sex not only to express pleasure and enhance the sexual experience but also to communicate her dislikes, set boundaries, and give instructions. She even began venturing into some dirty talk. Although our practice sessions usually ended in a lot of laughter, she was able to say things like "My pussy is so wet for you, Tim" and "I want your cock in my mouth" during her sexual encounters with Tim.

"He was so fucking blown away!" Jessica told me when she came to our last session with so much joy and confidence. "He was surprised and turned on. It made me feel so sexy!" I loved witnessing her blossoming with her sexual confidence. It's thrilling to see how sexual communication confidence positively contributes to my clients' lives in so many ways—not just in the bedroom. I believe that with education and practice, everyone can become a sexy confident communicator.

Good communication during sex is essential to long-term sexual satisfaction because you're the master of your own pleasure. Studies[49]

49. Elizabeth A. Babin, "An Examination of Predictors of Nonverbal and Verbal Communication of Pleasure During Sex and Sexual Satisfaction," *Journal of Social and Personal Relationships* 30, no. 3 (August 2012): 270–292, https://doi.org/10.1177/0265407512454523.

indicate that people who communicate during sex are more satisfied with their sex life. Micro sexual communication, which is communication during sex, can be verbal or nonverbal. People usually think nonverbal communication (e.g., showing you enjoy a sexual act by grabbing your partner harder or looking at them adoringly) is more natural and less awkward, but a mix of verbal and nonverbal communication usually works best because verbal communication allows for more clarity.[50] You can communicate your sexual likes and dislikes, express pleasure and displeasure, initiate sex, stop sex, and give directions for better sex.

Another hot thing to do during sex is give sexual compliments. I love receiving compliments during sex, and I'm sure most people do. That's why a praise kink exists. It could be a sweet compliment like "You look so pretty right now." One of my favorites is "Your ass tastes so good." This brings me to a prominent sexual communication concept: dirty talk. Good dirty talk is an art because it's not something anybody says in their daily life. Something like "Your cock is mine" is reserved for a passionate bedroom event only.

Let's start your micro sexual communication journey by rating your current sexual communication confidence from 1 to 10, where 1 means "I'm terrible at communicating during sex but ready to learn and improve" and 10 means "I'm extremely confident in my communication skills during sex. Anything I want, I say with ease, and anything I dislike, I sure as hell let them know!" Whatever your score is, it's all good. Once you have your score in mind, you can start honing your sexpertise in this chapter. I'm a fan of small but gradual improvements, so my goal is for you to improve your score by at least one point by the end of this chapter.

---

50. Heather Blunt-Vinti et al., "Show or Tell? Does Verbal and/or Nonverbal Sexual Communication Matter for Sexual Satisfaction?," *Journal of Sex & Marital Therapy* 45, no. 3 (April 2019): 206–217, https://doi.org/10.1080/0092623x.2018.1501446.

COMMUNICATION MISTAKES IN THE BEDROOM

Only asking about the climax: "Did you cum?" If your partner ever said that to you and you found yourself a little annoyed about it, you're not wrong (or alone). While the question might have been well-intentioned, it's bad sexual communication. That question is loaded with expectations of orgasm (people can still experience pleasure and connection without an orgasm), and it only allows for a *yes* or *no* answer. And let's real: The only viable answer here is *yes*; what's going to happen if you say *no*? A *no* response makes your partner die a little on the inside or get defensive about their sexual skills, so some people just choose to lie. Asking for sexual feedback should be more open-ended and empathetic. In this situation, you can instead ask, "How was it for you?" "What was your favorite part?" "How was that, baby?" or "What would you like me to do more or less next time?" Trust me, your partner will thank you for asking for sexual feedback in an open-minded way. It may also start a good conversation about the kind of sex you both want to explore.

Assuming someone's at fault: Another communication mistake that has caused countless issues is assuming someone is at fault when physical challenges arise. One client told me she asked, "What's wrong? Is it me?" when her husband lost his erection in the middle of sex and couldn't get hard again. She kept asking the same questions and he became extremely upset. When they came to my coaching session and told me what happened, I assured them that this is a very common communication mistake and it's easy to switch up the communicative response if something like that happens again. When men lose an erections during sex, they don't know what's wrong and are usually embarrassed and frustrated, so when a partner keeps asking what's wrong, it only makes the situation worse. Offering an alternative action for pleasure together is the best way to cope. Saying, "That's OK babe, can you go down on me?" "I'd love to take a break and cuddle," or "Let's give each other sensual massages" are just some examples of alternatives that don't need a hard dick. Don't try to have a full conversation about erectile dysfunction (ED) during a sexual encounter. It can be a very emotionally charged issue and should be discussed in a nonsexual context. During sex, try to move on and experience pleasure through other means that don't involve a hard penis. Don't try to pinpoint the cause of the physical challenge when you're both naked and sweaty!

Blaming: "I can't get hard because you didn't suck on it long enough." "I can't cum because you don't know how to fuck me." "I'm not wet because of you." These are real examples I've heard in my practice. Let me be up front: Blaming your partner is always terrible sexual communication. It can cause frustrations in the moment and resentment in the long run. It also shows that the blamer is insecure and will blame external factors for their problems. If you realize that you might have laid blame one or two times in the past, it's OK. Now is a good time to change and become more aware of negative communication behaviors. If you're dating a chronic blamer, then it's time for couple's counseling. It might be hard to unpack this issue by yourselves, so having a third-party professional can really help. If a sexual difficulty comes up, take a break or try other activities. Can't cum? Try incorporating a vibrator or a hand job. Not wet enough? Ask for oral sex or use your favorite lube. There is a creative solution for everything, so stop blaming and start working together to create a wonderful sex life.

Letting the silence linger: Not saying anything is also a big mistake. This is probably the one that most people make, and I totally understand why. Many of us were never taught what healthy sexual communication looks like in the bedroom. We learned from movies, TV, and porn, so I think it's safe to say we didn't grow up seeing examples of good bedroom conversations. Consequently, most people just choose to not say anything because it's easier and they don't want to rock the boat. So they don't speak up when the sex is bad, when it doesn't feel good, when it hurts, when it's too much, or when it's too little. Likewise, they also don't speak up when it's pleasurable, leaving their partners unsure and unaffirmed. Your partner can't read your mind and doesn't automatically know your preferences, so you need to speak up! Without proper communication, it's hard to have a satisfying sex life. And you deserve amazing sex!

Lying: How many people have lied about having an orgasm? I know I have. The act of orgasming itself is a form of communication. It says something about yourself and your sexual partner. Whether it's sexual satisfaction, a thumbs-up, or an affirmation that your partner is doing a good job, people usually create meaning behind their own and their partner's orgasms, which is why a lot of us choose to lie about it when we can't cum. However, faking an orgasm contributes to a negative loop because it doesn't allow your partner to improve and pleasure you better, which means you'll continue to have mediocre sex. Apart from cumming, people also lie about other things in bed. For example, they may say, "I love you" when they don't really mean it or "I've done it before" when they haven't. Lying can cause misunderstandings and build up resentment, so it's time to develop your sexual communication confidence and express yourself freely and accurately.

MICRO SEXUAL COMMUNICATION

Micro sexual communication is all the verbal and nonverbal communication that occurs *during* a sexual encounter. This includes everything from initiating sex to communicating pleasure, dislikes, and instructions. It also includes giving and receiving sexual feedback and expressing your boundaries. Of course, the ability to speak up for yourself during sex is much more associated with your sexual self-esteem and sexual knowledge. After reading previous chapters and doing the exercises I offered, my hope is that you feel more confident and capable in engaging in micro sexual communication as you read through this chapter.

***Trigger warning*: Content on unwanted sexual advances.** When I was in my twenties, I had poor sexual communication skills. I was great at flirting but not much else, and I certainly wasn't good at advocating for my own sexual safety and well-being. I was around eighteen when I had my first unwanted sexual encounter. I was tipsy and, like any insecure nineteen-year-old, wanted attention. I'd been texting with a guy who was a few years older than me about hanging out. He was attractive, confident, and a politician's son. He came to pick me up in his white BMW two-seater. In my mind, I just wanted to hang out and flirt, but in his mind, he wanted to fuck. In retrospect, all I could think was that I should have known better.

After a few attempts to take me to his bed, I gave in. Not only that, but *I performed*. I'm sure it was so fucking hot for him. I didn't know how to advocate for myself, and he took advantage of my insecurity and lack of self-esteem. When we were done—when *he* was done (of course I didn't cum)—he told me to put my clothes on and that he would drop me off because he had to wake up early the next day. In the car, he held my hand, but we said nothing. He dropped me off, and we never talked again. I felt disgusted afterward but was also too tired to stay awake and beat myself up. I woke up the next day thinking I should have said something, should have been sterner, should have communicated up front that I wasn't looking for sex, but—shoulda, woulda, coulda—I told myself to just forget about it.

Micro sexual communication is also about advocating for your own physical and emotional safety. The ability to stand up for yourself is a key part of sexual empowerment. Sexual initiation is an attempt to have consensual sex with someone. For this attempt to be successful, consent must be asked for and given freely. Here's a fun acronym to remember: FRIES (also one of my favorite food items). Proper consent is **f**reely given (they're not forced), **r**eversible (they're allowed to change their mind), **i**nformed (they know what they're doing), **e**nthusiastic (it's a fuck yeah), and **s**pecific (they agree to certain activities within parameters; for example, just because I said yes to making out doesn't mean I want to have penetrative sex). Making sure that both partners (or more) are always enthusiastic and consenting is key. Even though saying *no* might not be easy for some of us, hesitance should always be taken as a *no*.

SEXUAL INITIATION FOR COUPLES

There's no one-size-fits-all approach to sexual initiation. There are many strategies people use that are based on various factors like age, relationship status, closeness, sexual orientation, past experience, emotional intimacy level, the kind of sex being initiated, hormones, physical health, and so on. What works for one person may not work for another. You need to decide what works for you and your partner.

Sexual initiation often speaks louder than words. If you're in a long-term relationship, you know what I'm talking about. When your partner hasn't initiated sex for a long time, it can feel like you're not desirable. Even if you just started dating, initiating sex can be a type of love language (when it's wanted). The act of initiation (or the lack thereof) can communicate much about the current health of a relationship. When people are unhappy and resentful, they don't have the desire to initiate sex and the thought of it can make them feel disgusted. By contrast, when they feel emotionally connected and safe, and they have passion for each other, sexual initiation happens regularly (unless you're asexual).

Let me be clear about something, though: Regular doesn't mean every day. Again, it means different things for different people. For some, it might be four times a week. For others, it might be four times a month. It's whatever you desire. But the initiation part shouldn't be extremely difficult if the relationship is healthy.

Direct + Verbal Initiation = "Wanna Fuck?"

As a sex educator, I always encourage people to try direct verbal communication when they want to initiate sex because it provides the most clarity. There are various intensity levels, based on how dirty you want to be and how close you feel to your sexual partner, that range from "Would you like to have sex with me?" to "I'd like to ride you tonight; would you like that?" Oh yeah, verbal communication is sexy.

"That's such a buzzkill," a student once said in my class. It's only a buzzkill if you're uncomfortable with sexual communication. For most skilled and confident lovers, direct asks are so fucking hot. I learned this a long time ago the very first time someone was confidently up front with me. I remember being in a rooftop bar in Paris and flirting with a guy. The vibe was amazing and there was plenty of flirting. He looked at me adoringly, and I kept touching his hand and tapping his shoulder. As the bar was closing, he leaned over real close and whispered, "You want to fuck me, don't you?" OMG, I had no idea how hot that would be until someone directly asked me.

"Fuck yeah, I do," I smiled. And the rest of the night was fireworks.

Ever since then, I've been up front about my sexual desire for someone. If I want to fuck you, I make sure you know about it. This type of initiation is easier if you're confident and extroverted, and it will be more successful if your partner has been giving you cues of their sexual desires for you. What if they say, "No, I don't want to have sex with you"? So what? People say *no* all the time for all kinds of things. You can just reply, "That's all right. I had a great time chatting with you." Rejection is not the end of the world.

For couples who like to baby talk (referring to each other endearingly), this can be as direct as saying, "Sexy time tonight, baby?" Sexting is another great way to prime your partner before you get it on. It's so sexy to see sexts like "can't wait to fuck your brains out tonight ;-)" or "thinking of you and I'm so wet, should we spend tomorrow morning in bed?" All these fun strategies are great when there's already intimacy and closeness in the relationship.

Indirect + Verbal Initiation = "Sweet Potato!"

For fun couples who enjoy a playful and lighthearted way to get it on, try creating silly code words that communicate your desire to initiate sex, such as *sweet potato* or *coloring book*. This is a great initiation technique for couples who have children or live with other people—as well as for people who are more introverted with a playful personality. Using sarcasm can also be a good indirect verbal initiation method: "Oh, right, I'm not at all horny" or "Not sure if my hard-on is because I'm so turned on by you or I'm just cold." If you have that kind of rapport in your relationship—where there's a lot of joking, sarcasm, and banter—then this strategy can work really well.

Giving compliments is another indirect verbal strategy. You can opt for compliments that are more suggestive like "Your butt looks extra sexy today" or "You look *good* in those sweatpants, babe." This is a great strategy for all couples, whether you've been dating a few months or many years. Make sure that the compliments are about them and not what they can do for you. For example, "You're so good at washing dishes" is *not* a sexy compliment and won't work as sexual initiation. In general, though, compliments are wonderful at keeping a relationship joyful and positive, so make sure you give them regularly.

Direct + Nonverbal = *Sliding the Hand Down the Pants*

My husband and I often use this initiation strategy. He's more of a non-verbal guy, but I'm teaching him to become more verbal because I have a soft spot for dirty talk. He loves it when I casually play with his cock to initiate sex, whether we're watching TV, doing chores, or driving somewhere. (Warning: This last one can be dangerous, so do it at your own risk.) Likewise, he'll massage my breasts or try to lift up my dress to caress my legs and pubic area to communicate that he's horny. We also love outdoor sex, so when we go hiking, he'll put my hand on his dick over his pants and tell me he wants to get it on.

This strategy works best for long-term couples or if you've been together at least six months and feel very comfortable with each other's sexual initiation and communication styles. I do not recommend this approach for new couples or if you're still in the early dating stage because it may feel like you're doing unsolicited touching or giving unwanted sexual advances, which is the opposite of sexy. It's gross.

Direct nonverbal initiation doesn't have to involve touch, though. You can also use props. For music lovers who like to communicate and express their horniness through sexy sounds, try creating a sex playlist to hint to your partner that you're turned on and want to turn up the heat. Sex toys can also be helpful in this situation. For example, a friend will pick up a sex toy, show it to her husband, and he immediately knows she wants some sexy time. These strategies are great for long-term couples who already have an established understanding of each other's initiation styles. For newer couples, make sure you communicate your desire to initiate sex this way first, then ask how they feel about it. If they're down, then awesome! Have fun!

Indirect + Nonverbal = Hinting My Way Into You

This is a slow-burn strategy where you try to engage in nonverbal activities to help set the mood and subtly express your sexual desire. Examples include a shoulder massage and other acts of service, such as doing the dishes and preparing a relaxing bath. The downside of this strategy is that your sexual partner may not notice that you're hinting at an opportunity for sexual connection; they may miss it completely or just take it as a simple act of love and nothing more. For some people, indirect seduction may work. Think of sexy lingerie or lighting candles. It can also involve touch, such as hand holding or running your fingers through your partner's hair. Indirect nonverbal initiation can be romantic and sweet, and it can be used by both new and long-term couples. It's important that you read the cues, though. If your partner hesitates or seems uncomfortable, that should be read as a *no*, and you shouldn't pursue further. Try to have a conversation about sexual initiation styles in a nonsexual context to uncover what your partner prefers and to share what you like.

THE DON'TS OF SEXUAL INITIATION

- **Don't threaten to end the relationship or cheat on your partner as a sexual initiation technique. Saying things like "If you don't fuck me, I guess it's over" or "You left me no choice; if I can't have sex with you, then I'll go have sex with someone else" is terrible sexual communication and extremely hurtful.**
- **Don't try to initiate sex with someone who's too drunk or too high. It's immoral and the consequences can be grave.**
- **Don't get upset and make negative comments with your partner for rejecting your sexual advances. If their rejections occur frequently and it's hurtful to you, bring it up in a nonsexual context.**
- **Don't ask for sexual things in an arrogant way like "Can you suck my dick?"**
- **Don't initiate with indifference or a lack of effort, like "Ugh, I guess I can give you a hand job before I go to bed" or "Are we having sex or what? I'm already tired." If you're initiating sex, make sure you express yourself with enthusiasm. Sex is the most pleasurable when both people put in the effort.**

WHAT CAN I SAY IN BED?

During sex, you can express all kinds of things through verbal communication. For example, after giving your partner oral, you can ask, "Can I put my finger inside you?" or "Can I eat your ass?" Always make sure you ask for and receive consent before moving on to the next sexual act. You can communicate pleasure ("Oh, that feels good, baby" or "Ah! You're making me cum"), you can communicate discomfort ("Um, that hurts" or "Ow! That was too rough"), you can communicate likes and dislikes ("I love it when you suck on my nipples" or "I don't like my ears licked"), you can give instructions ("Slower, baby" or "Can you use more lube?"), and you can give compliments ("Your moan is so sexy" or "I love watching your hot, naked body"). If verbalizing your thoughts and feelings in bed isn't so much your thing, nonverbal communication can still be effective. Keep in mind that verbal communication can provide more clarity to your sexual partner, so I'd recommend you try confidence practices to grow your sexual communication confidence.

DIRTY TALK

Sex is like a baked potato: It can be bland, or it can be loaded with yummy toppings. Dirty talk is like one of those toppings on a loaded baked potato. It makes sex even more delicious! In short, dirty talk encompasses verbal messages that are taboo, derogatory (to a varying degree), and often not politically correct. A lot of things said as dirty talk are context specific and not something you would ever say outside that context. For comparison, "I love having sex with you" is an affirmation, but "I love having your throbbing cock inside my pussy" is dirty talk.

Studies[51] show that people with higher sexual self-esteem tend to engage in dirty talk more frequently. That makes sense since sexual self-esteem is very much intertwined with communication confidence. If you feel like you deserve pleasure and are self-assured in your sexuality, then you're going to have more room to play and more mental capacity

---

51. Margaret Bennett, "Talk Dirty to Me: An Examination of the Effects of Communication During Sexual Activity on Relational Outcomes for Young Adults Beginning Romantic Relationships" (PhD diss., University of Connecticut, 2019), 1–113, https://digitalcommons.lib.uconn.edu/dissertations/2209/.

to experiment with something like dirty talk. Remember, it's best to ask your partner how they feel about dirty talk to gauge their interest and level of intensity. Just like most communication concepts, you can adjust the level of intensity to your liking, from sexy and raunchy to nasty! The following are five common types of dirty talk.

Compliments: Most people love receiving compliments in bed, especially when it's charged with sexual energy and the "taboo-ness" of dirty talk. You can compliment someone's skills and the way they look, feel, taste, and smell. Compliments can enhance the sexual experience, create a stronger bond between partners, and increase the sexual self-esteem level for the receiver. Examples include "Your body is fucking amazing," "Your cock/pussy tastes so good," and "You're so good at riding daddy."

Narration: Hearing your lover use a sexy voice to narrate what's going on in bed can really turn up the heat. It can be a short sentence or a whole movie, depending on the skills of the narrator who uses vivid and descriptive language to create more tension and enhance the sexual encounter. My friend Jen is a narrator. She likes to narrate dirty shit that's going on in the moment or every sexy thing she sees. She'd say things like "Your big cock is so veiny, and it was throbbing in my mouth," "Oh, I love seeing your cock deep inside me; it feels so warm and hard," and "You're a master at eating my pussy; flicking your tongue up and down pleasuring my clit is my favorite morning ritual." *That's narrating.* This is, admittedly, a very difficult skill. Personally, when I have sex, I'm so focused on sensations that it's hard for me to narrate, but some lovers do it so well, and it's fucking hot when they can.

Direction: Giving directions to your sexual partner is probably one of the most used dirty talk categories because it feels natural to assert yourself in a sexual way by telling someone what to do. If you enjoy power dynamics, particularly if you like being the person with more domineering energy, you'll love doing this form of dirty talk. Examples include "I want to see your face deep in my pussy," "Fuck me harder," "Come suck on my nipples," "Pull my hair and fuck me hard," "Shoot a load in my mouth," and "Get my cock deep down your throat."

Ownership/Submission: This is probably the least politically correct category of dirty talk. Saying you own someone or that they're your slave isn't something you should *ever* say outside a consensual sexual context. Lovers who enjoy varying power dynamics of dom/sub and master/slave find this type of dirty talk natural and of course very hot! You can say, "This cock/pussy is mine," "You're my sex slave," "I'm your dirty slut," "Your body is mine and only mine," "I'm wearing this collar just for you," "Take my pussy/cock, I'm all yours," "Your cum is mine; hold it until I say you can cum," and "I own your mouth, so put this cock deep down your throat, you dirty whore."

Questions: This is a great category for everyone, from beginner to advanced dirty talkers. All lovers can benefit from asking sexy dirty questions as it enhances the sexual experience and turns up the heat even more. It's also a great way to help your partner—who might not be as fluent in dirty talk—start doing it by answering your questions. You can ask anything that you find hot, such as "How does my wet pussy feel, daddy?" "Do you know how hard I am for you right now?" "Do you want me to fuck you harder?" "How does it feel to have my hard cock inside you?" "Who's a good girl/boy?" and "What do you want me to do with your cock?"

Don't forget to have a conversation about dirty talk before you actually engage and practice it. It might bring up negative memories, or your partner may find it completely disgusting. This is why it's so important to ask first before you do it. Early in the dating relationship, you should ask, "How do you feel about dirty talk?" so you know before your first time having sex!

THE THINGS YOU SHOW IN BED (NONVERBAL COMMUNICATION)

Nonverbal expressions are usually seen as less awkward and not so threatening during sex. A study found women are less likely to verbally communicate in bed to partner with fragile masculinity[52]. Another study found both men and women prefer using facial expressions and body movements to communicate during sex.[53] Nonverbal expressions are a key factor in any successful sexual encounter, be it showing you're into it with your face, grabbing your partner harder, or connecting deeply with your partner by gazing in their eyes. Nonverbal expressions allow you to authentically communicate with your eyes, face, body, and touch.

You can express consent nonverbally as long as it's clear and enthusiastic. You can maintain eye contact, smile, kiss, nod *yes*, and guide your partner's hand onto your body. For example, if I'm making deep eye contact with you while licking and biting my lip . . . oh yeah, I want to get it on. Many people express pleasure by moaning (a form of nonverbal communication called *paralinguistics* because you're just making sounds and not verbalizing messages). People love hearing their partner moan because it's an affirmation that they're doing a good job. Full disclosure: I'm a loud moaner. It's how I get all that pent-up energy out. In the past, I've dated people who shushed me during sex, which made me feel so ashamed of myself. With my current partner, I told him from the beginning that I'm wild during sex and do not need shushing. He supports me 100 percent and enjoys my animalistic expression, so that makes sex even more amazing.

---

52. Audrey Lutmer and Alicia M. Walker, "Patterns of Verbal and Nonverbal Communication during Sex," *Archives of Sexual Behavior* 53, no. 4 (April 2024): 1449–1462, https://pubmed.ncbi.nlm.nih.gov/38361172/.
53. Blunt-Vinti, "Show or Tell?," 206–217.

Pleasure is often expressed through body language. Many women squirm when they're about to have an orgasm and their pelvic area pushes up a bit before they squirt. Lots of people dig their fingers and nails into their partner's skin to show pleasure. When you like something your partner is doing, you might use your hand to reinforce the act (e.g., when my partner goes down on me, I use my hand to gently push his head down and play with his hair to express that I really like it). Likewise, expressing discomfort through nonverbal expressions is also common. Pulling your body away, closing your legs, or making a painful facial expression can all communicate displeasure or dislike. Your sexual partner is constantly talking to you through their body language, so be a great lover and spend time learning how to read these cues.

SEXUAL EXPRESSION STYLE

One of my friends moans so loudly when she orgasms that her neighbor once left her a note asking her to shut the hell up. On the other hand, I have a client who is very quiet and tense when he has sex. Which are you? Or maybe you're somewhere in the middle? Whatever your current sexual expression style (SES), rest assured that you're normal and can change if you desire.

There are four types of SES: animalistic, serene, tense, and doubtful. I have an animalistic expression. That means I'm uninhibited, loud, and probably look weird when I orgasm, but I don't care. I bite and scratch and grab pretty aggressively when I experience pleasure. But I wasn't always animalistic. Once upon a time, I was doubtful and wasn't sure how I should express myself during sex. I was worried about how to moan so I sound sexy and how to arch my back so my date would think I was hot. I was filled with uncertainty. Those days are long gone, but I wonder how many of us are still in a similar phase?

Let's identify your current style and which style you may want to strive for as you embark on your journey of sexual liberation.

Animalistic (high energy, uninhibited) • Upbeat, loud, and high-energy lovers who express themselves freely without any doubts or shame	Tense (high energy, inhibited) • Loud and high-energy lovers who express themselves in a choreographic manner and in limiting ways
Serene (gentle energy, uninhibited) • Sensual, gentle, and calm lovers who express themselves freely without any doubts and shame	Doubtful (gentle energy, inhibited) • Awkward lovers who express themselves with uncertainty and nervousness

PILLOW TALK

It's great to talk about lovey-dovey things after sex so you can maximize all the feel-good hormones rushing through you after great sex and orgasms. If you want to build trust, a stronger bond,[54] and feelings of closeness within a relationship, you should consider doing postcoital disclosures, otherwise known as pillow talk, otherwise known as having a positive conversation after sexual activity. Research[55] has found that couples who engage in pillow talk report higher levels of relationship satisfaction. Perhaps rushing to do something else after sex that's not meaningful, like getting on the phone to look at social media or watching TV, sends the message that you just wanted sexual gratification—not sexual connection—which can hurt the relationship. Spend time with your partner in bed for at least ten minutes after sex to wind down together and have loving conversations. Use this list to guide you!

- **"How was it, baby?"**
- **"How was it when I [insert action]?"**

---

54. Amanda Denes, "Pillow Talk: Exploring Disclosures After Sexual Activity," *Western Journal of Communication* 76, no. 2 (March 2012): 91–108, https://doi.org/10.1080/10570314.2011.651253.

55. Amanda Denes, "Gene X Environment Interactions and Pillow Talk: Investigating the Associations Among the OXTR Gene, Orgasm, Post-Sex Communication, and Relationship Satisfaction in Young Adult Relationships," *Communication Studies* 72, no. 1 (August 2020): 68–65, https://doi.org/10.1080/10510974.2020.1807373.

- **Praise your partner and the sex you just enjoyed together.**
- **Express how much you love your partner and their positive qualities.**
- **"What were some positive moments for you this week?"**
- **"What are you manifesting right now in your life?"**
- **"How do you feel about exploring more of what we just did?" (if you just tried something new)**
- **"Why do you think our relationship works so well?"**
- **"What are some qualities of mine that you really love?"**
- **"What would you like to do for our date night this/next week?"**
- **"What's a positive sexual memory you have of us from the past few months?"**

POST-SEX ETIQUETTE

Here are a few things you should do after sex as a great and responsible lover:

1. **Offer the "niceties" (e.g., water, wet wipes, candy).**
2. **Ask how it was for them!**
3. **Stay in bed, cuddle, and chat for at least ten minutes (unless it's a quickie).**
4. **Want to be extra sweet? Offer a little massage after sex.**
5. **Want to be sensual? Take a warm bath together.**
6. **If it's casual sex, you should still treat your partner with respect! Maybe you're not staying overnight, but make sure you do the first two ideas above, and then text to thank them for a good time.**

Quite a journey, huh? Micro sexual communication is essential in our sexual well-being, so it's worth taking time to do it and improve it.

I want to invite you to reflect on all the information you've just learned and see whether your sexual communication confidence score has gone up by at least one point from all this knowledge. I truly believe that after processing everything you've learned thus far, you will feel more assured and empowered as a sexual being!

Chapter 8

Sex Tech and Sex Tools

A great sext is all about anticipation . . . kind of like foreplay.

—Dr. Emily Morse

Sex and technology have always been besties—through the good, the bad, and the crazy. (Have you heard of the Orgasmatron 3000 washing machine that women can ride on top of?!) The birth of the internet also brought about the birth of porn sites. With the development of electric tools? We got vibrators and other sex toys. With the push of e-commerce? People started selling dildos and butt plugs online. With the advancement of smartphones? We all began sexting with photos, videos, GIFs, and memes. And it's not stopping there. With advanced technology and artificial intelligence, we got VR porn and AI sex robots[56] that can cum on command and change their demeanors based on the user!

It seems like technology and sex is an everlasting relationship that will continue forward for as long as humans are alive. As someone who loves technology, I support technological advancements that bring connection, pleasure, education, and entertainment to people. I agree that we need strong regulations for safe tools and ethical considerations for

56. Slutever, "Meet Harmony the Sex Robot," video, posted March 14, 2018, by VICE TV, YouTube, www.youtube.com/watch?v=orBH_Qnw3eY.

all products and developments, but consumers must also use this tech and these tools mindfully. They need to do their own research when purchasing a product or service because, like anything else in life, there are good and bad ones.

I've seen so many people use sex tech mindlessly. One friend is so addicted to sexting with an online content creator that he doesn't spend much time developing and maintaining relationships in real life. He always complains, "It's so hard to date a girl in my city."

One time, I asked him, "So who's the girl that you said you'll go home and talk to last night after we went to the gym?"

He responded, "Oh, that's Crystal. She's an online sexy content creator, but I feel like we have a thing, you know? I don't mind paying her to sext with me. Maybe I'm helping her with the college fund."

After he showed me their sext/text conversation, which seemed pretty standard for such a transactional relationship, I told him the truth. "Hey, listen. I don't think the relationship you're developing with her is going anywhere. It's for instant comfort and sexual gratification. It's transactional, which is fine in moderation because it's your prerogative, but she's not interested in becoming your girlfriend. And she won't be helping you out if you lose your job or can't pay her. I just want to be real with you."

Do you have a friend, family member, or partner who might be addicted to some kind of sex tech? If left unchecked, it can become quite a challenge to recover from. One client is a self-proclaimed "vibrator addict" and has used a vibrator daily for the last ten years. She and her husband came to a coaching session to reinvigorate their passion for each other because it had grown dry and dull. When I saw them, they hadn't had sex in almost three years. He blamed her vibrator for everything, but is a sex tool the root cause? Or is it because they both have been neglecting their sexual connection? Lots of people use sex toys to enhance their sex lives and their connection as a couple, so why couldn't they?

In this chapter, I'll cover different types of sex tech, toys, and tools—and how they influence our sexual well-being, relational development, and relationship enhancement. I want to note that I'm focusing on the interpersonal aspects of sex tech in this chapter. For a more comprehensive discussion of porn, see Chapter 10.

SEXTING

"Hey, handsome 🔥 I thought of you and my pussy is wet 💦 all over my office chair."

Of course, when I talk about sexting, I mean *consensual* sexting. I do not condone unsolicited sexting to strangers—just so we're on the same page. Sexting is not a new phenomenon. Rumor has it that Napoleon wrote a note to his lover Empress Josephine saying, "I'm returning in three days. Don't wash," implying he wanted to smell the natural scent of her pussy when he returned from battle. In a way, that was an early form of sexting.

Even though humans have always engaged in this type of communication, sexting became a popular cultural phenomenon around the world in the twenty-first century with the rise of smartphones, and it's now pretty universal. I've lived in Thailand, Finland, and the United States, and I've talked to people from around the world; I know we all sext. Whether you're in a small American town or a big city in South Korea, someone you know is sexting. In fact, texting is Gen Z's most common and preferred method of communication[57]

Should you send a sexy pic of yourself in lingerie or write about how you're touching yourself in bed? Should you write suggestively or vividly?

---

57. Melanie Gaboriault, "What I've Learned About the New Era of Communication from my Gen Z Kids," *Fast Company*, December 11, 2022, https://www.fastcompany.com/90819951/what-ive-learned-about-the-new-era-of-communication-from-my-gen-z-kids.

How should you prime your date or partner that you're about to send a NSFW video? I love sexting, but there are definitely unspoken rules everyone should know—that I'm going to share in this chapter.

Sexting isn't just for younger people; older people do it too. One survey[58] indicated that more than half of all participants over 57 years old had done it during the previous year. Research[59] also indicates same-sex couples are five times more likely to sext than heterosexual couples. In heterosexual dating, it's been found that women are more likely to sext than men[60] (but trust me when I say we don't like unsolicited dick pics and sexual messages). Women tend to sext within their romantic relationships, whereas men are also down to sext with casual and online partners. Men are also more likely to enjoy visual stimuli, such as sexy and nude pics. Studies[61] have also confirmed that sexting is great for long-term couples; it increases the level of sexual satisfaction and improves romantic relationships. It's also such a great way to maintain sexual intimacy for long-distance couples. Not only is it great for committed relationships, it's also linked to self-empowerment. Personally, when I sext my husband, I feel like a badass sexual goddess. It's a fun and useful practice.

It's important to note that sexting is legal between *consenting adults*. Sending unsolicited sexts to strangers is gross—and illegal if either party is under 18. There are far too many cases where teens' nudes are leaked

---

58. Stacy Tessler Lindau et al., "A Study of Sexuality and Health Among Older Adults in the United States," *New England Journal of Medicine* 357, no. 8 (August 2007): 762–774, https://doi.org/10.1056/nejmoa067423.

59. Deborah Gordon-Messer et al., "Sexting Among Young Adults," *Journal of Adolescent Health* 52, no. 3 (March 2013): 301–306, https://doi.org/10.1016/j.jadohealth.2012.05.013.

60. Pamela Paul, "He Sexts, She Sexts More, Report Says," *New York Times*, July 15, 2011, www.nytimes.com/2011/07/17/fashion/women-are-more-likely-to-sext-than-men-study-says-studied.html?_r=1&src=recg.

61. Jia Jian Tin et al., "Potential Benefits of Sexting Among Long-term Monogamous Romantic Partners," *Journal of Counseling Sexology & Sexual Wellness: Research, Practice, and Education* 3, no. 2 (January 2022): 30–38, https://doi.org/10.34296/03021053.

(or threatened to be leaked), which unfortunately led to suicide[62]. It's better to advise your teenage kids, siblings, cousins, and friends to wait until they're adults and in a healthy relationship before they engage in sexting. However, the truth is that a lot of high schoolers are sexting and sending sexy pics to their boyfriends and girlfriends, even if the adults in their lives say, "Don't do it, it's dangerous," which is why it's so important to highlight safety when it comes to these matters.

Here are some tips to keep everyone safe when engaging in sexting:

1. **Use an app or function that makes your message disappear (but know that you still run the risk of people taking screenshots of it).**

2. **Don't send a pic with your face in it unless you're in a committed relationship and 100 percent trust your partner.**

3. **Don't sext a completely nude picture. You can still send a sexy pic without full nudity.**

I think sexting is so much fun (when done right), but it's not everybody's cup of tea. I remember trying to sext someone I went on a date with, but his responses just flat-out shut it down. I get it. Not everyone finds it sexy or wants to engage with it, and some people just don't think they're "good at it," so they'd rather not sext at all. For those of you who are curious and potentially want to get better at it, know that you totally can. It's a skill, not a trait. It's not like someone was born to be a sexter. Everyone, even if you think you're super awkward, can learn to be good at sexting.

There are many types of communication that fall under the sexting umbrella, including sexual messages, sexy photos and videos, sexual memes and GIFs, porn clips, audio porn and ASMR clips, links to erotica, emojis, and voice notes of dirty talk or moaning. Whatever you prefer and whatever your level of comfort is, there is a method of sexting that's

---

62. Rikki Schlott, "Parents Reveal Teen Sons Committed Suicide After Being 'Sextorted': 'This Is Terrorism,'" *New York Post*, August 30, 2023, nypost.com/2023/08/30/parents-reveal-teen-sons-committed-suicide-after-sextortion/.

perfect for you. Should you send a sexy lingerie pic or a dirty message? Why not both?! If you're comfortable, sending both can enhance the sexting experience. A lot of people, not just men, are stimulated visually (me included), yet some prefer text messages and using their imagination, so sending both can cover all your bases.

How should you prime your date or partner that you want to sext with them? If it's a new partner or someone you just started dating, ask how they feel about sexting to gauge their thoughts and interest level. If they have a positive view of it, next time you want to sext, you can first ask, "Would you like to see a sexy pic of me after my gym session? ;-)" Then gauge the interest from there. If you've been dating for a bit, you can also enact a "green, yellow, red rule" where you can send a code emoji like *fire*. If they send green back, then it means they're good to receive some NSFW stuff. If they send yellow, it can mean they'll be ready soon (e.g., after five minutes). Red obviously means not right now. This rule is great because it allows for two people to be active participants in the process.

What about tips for appropriate sexting? The answer to this is honestly so individualized. I love nasty shit, but a lot of my friends totally dislike it and their version of sexting is, to me, regular flirting. The general rule of thumb is that it must be consensual, focused on building anticipation and connection (not just to show off), and fun! Now let's look at a few different categories of sexting and see which ones are best for you and your partner.

Sexting Categories and Levels of Intensity

MESSAGES

Just like dirty talk, there are many levels and types of messages you can send. Sexting may seem hard at first, especially if you don't feel confident in your sexual communication skills, but because you're not physically together, you're able to craft perfectly sexy messages that IRL sex just doesn't allow. Should you write suggestively or vividly? It's entirely up to you. Recall the dirty talk categories: compliments, narration, direction, ownership/submission, and questions. You can also use any of these in sexting. Here are some examples with varying levels of heat:

- **Mild and cheeky: "Did you miss me today? What would you do to me right now?**
- **Medium spice: "I'd like to slowly take your clothes off and lick every part of your body. Kiss your neck, devour your nipples, and oh would you like to hear what I want to do with your pussy?"**
- **Hot damn!: "I'll put your cock deep down my throat and gag on it while I play with your balls. Then I'll suck on your balls and make your cock even harder. I want you to cum on my face!"**

PHOTOS

In some cases, a picture is absolutely worth a thousand words. A lot of people like getting sexy pics from their dates or partners. I know I do! So what's a good pic to send? Well, let's take a look at the varying levels of heat:

- **Mild and cheeky: Send a pic of you looking sexy—something like a shirtless pic (men) or a lingerie/underwear pic (women). A kissy face is also flirty and a good start for sexting. A suggestive photo of an object is also good, such as a pic of handcuffs, a blindfold, other sex toys, or a dress you're about to wear on a date.**
- **Medium spice: Send a dick pic (men) or topless pic (women), with or without your face (up to you and your trust level). Include a variety of poses. Make sure you groom before you send the dick pic!**
- **Hot damn!: Send a full-frontal, fully nude pic with or without your face. Maybe a pic of you cumming from masturbation, fully nude and from behind (maybe show you're playing with your butthole if that's the vibe), dick pics with cum, or a wet kitty pic.**

VIDEOS

If a picture is worth a thousand words, then a video is worth a million. However, videos can be hit or miss for some people. I've talked to many people who love receiving masturbation videos from someone they're dating or their long-term partner, but a few people have said, "Eww, no, that's gross." To each their own, I guess, but you know me by now—I love it.

- **Mild and cheeky: Send a short, ten-second video of you touching parts of your body (not the genitals). For men, this could be a video of you playing with your dick on top of your pants. For women, it could be a video of you playing with your breasts on top of your clothes or a quick peek of your naked butt from behind.**
- **Medium spice: Send a 15- to 30-second video of you touching your naked body, which can briefly include your genitals (as a tease). For women, this could be playing with your bare breasts and nipples or putting a vibrator on your clit. For men, it could be a video of you playing with your dick and balls. Maybe also show your abs and chest while playing with your nipples.**
- **Hot damn!: Send a full masturbation video (with or without face), complete with cum at the end. Since people love seeing their partner cum, the ending must be included; it's the grand finale! The video can be from the beginning of your solo session or maybe from the middle or toward the end so you can show the cum shot/orgasm.**

OTHER CATEGORIES

Other categories of sexting that are less popular—but still poppin'—are sending memes and GIFs. These can be subtle and suggestive, like a meme of someone licking a Popsicle, or they can be very sexual, like full-blown nude GIFs.

Porn, audio porn, and ASMR clips are perfect when you want to set the mood or maybe share something you want to do in real life later. Before sending any clips, though, make sure you ask for a green light first. Many people have their messages connected to their computers. You might accidentally send a porn video to your partner while they're giving a presentation in class or sharing their screen in a business meeting. You never know. In addition, don't just send clips without context. Explain briefly why you're sending it, so your partner can understand. For example, you may send an anal sex clip and say, "I've fantasized about us doing this. What do you think? ;-)" You can also send audio porn and say, "This makes me think of you," or you can send ASMR of oral sex and say, "This is what I'm doing to you tonight." So many choices!

Any literature enthusiasts in the house? Erotica excerpts are great for people who love reading and creating a slow-simmering sexual tension. It can be an amazing way to build sexual connection slowly and more mindfully without being distracted by provocative visuals or sounds. Copy, paste, and send the parts that you find really hot. These excerpts can help tune your partner into your sexual desires and spark sexual exchanges.

A less personal way of sexting, but one that is definitely easier, is simply sending emojis. You can send all kinds of suggestive emojis to initiate or respond to your partner's sexts. If you're not yet "good with words," this might be an easy way to start—but make sure you graduate quickly to other categories. Experienced sexters won't want to keep sexting with someone who only knows how to communicate through emojis.

Finally, sending a voice note where you say something sexy like, "Thinking of you eating me out last night" or "Can't wait to see you devour my pussy tonight" can be a huge turn-on for the receiver.

Adding one of these categories of sexting to your relationship can enhance your sex life, sexual self-esteem, and connection with your partner. Satisfaction guaranteed.

The Dos And Don'ts Of Sexting

DOS:

- **Ask for a green light before you start sexting.**
- **Experiment with different categories and techniques of sexting to see which ones work best for you and your partner.**
- **Approach it with playfulness.**
- **Only send pics you're comfortable with.**
- **Explore sexting with an open mind because you never know what your partner is going to send back!**

DON'TS:

- **Send nudes with your face in it when you don't know the other person that well.**
- **Send unsolicited pics and videos.**
- **Use the same message over and over.**
- **Judge your partner negatively if their sexting game isn't strong. (It takes practice!)**
- **Try to force someone to send you nudes or sext with you. (Some people are really not ready or are absolutely against it.)**

CYBERSEX

Technically, you can have sex with people online without even knowing their real name or seeing their real face. Cybersex describes any sexual encounter in which two or more people are "having a sexual experience" online or through a video call. Many sites offer these opportunities—usually for men. Interestingly, only about 10 percent of users of these platforms (not creators) are women.

Cybersex has been steadily becoming more prominent and popular, but there was a drastic increase during and after the COVID-19 pandemic[63] because it is an effective way for online creators to create income. In 2023, one of the biggest sites for online sex work reported having more than 100 million users and billions of dollars in revenue[64]. Keep in mind, though, that not all cybersex is between a creator and a client. Many times, it's between lovers, daters, long-distance partners, and

63. Valeria Rubattu et al., "'Cam Girls and Adult Performers Are Enjoying a Boom in Business': The Reportage on the Pandemic Impact on Virtual Sex Work," *Social Sciences* 12, no. 2 (January 2023): 62, https://doi.org/10.3390/socsci12020062.
64. Todd Spangler, "OnlyFans Payments Surged to Record $6.6 Billion in 2023, Up 19%," *Variety*, September 6, 2024, https://variety.com/2024/digital/news/onlyfans-payments-2023-financials-revenue-creator-earnings-1236135425/.

long-term couples. For couples in long-distance relationships, cybersex allows them to stay intimate and sexually connected. Research[65] found that cybersex is beneficial for these couples, but they still experience challenges like initiation (i.e., figuring out who's starting it) and timing (i.e., determining when it's appropriate). I know many of us, myself included, want to sext and cybersex our partner when they're away. For example, when my husband recently went out of town, I made sure we masturbated together on FaceTime before we went to bed. I like to prop my phone on the side table so he can see my breasts and body movement but not my face.

Activities like cybersex and sexting are amazing ways technology can help us find novelty and excitement in our sexual relationships. However, I want to note that we still live in a world with bad people. I had one student tell me that the person she was dating for a couple months screenshotted their cybersex session and shared it on Snapchat. She learned about it because she had a mutual friend who saw the post and told her about it. She broke up with him after a long text chain back and forth with him apologizing but also saying, "I don't know why it's a big deal. People know we're dating." All this to say that you need to be mindful when participating in sexy activities online. Use good judgment to determine safe practices, knowing that sometimes people can still be insensitive and disrespectful even with the right precautions. Ultimately, as safe as you think you're being, you still run the risk of meeting assholes who will use your photos to their advantage. Remember though: It's never your fault when someone like that shares photos without your permission.

65. Carman Neustaedter and Saul Greenberg, "Intimacy in Long-Distance Relationships Over Video Chat," *Proceedings of the SIGCHI Conference on Human Factors in Computing Systems* (May 2012): 753–762, https://doi.org/10.1145/2207676.2207785.

SEX TOOLS AND SEX TOYS

Thirty thousand years old! That's the age of the oldest sex toy that's been discovered: a dildo-shaped baton from the Upper Paleolithic period.[66] Hallie Lieberman, a leading scholar of sex toys whom I had the pleasure of interviewing on *LuvBites by Dr. Tara*, told me all about the early inventions of toys for fun, pleasure, excitement, and "other" (some just exist without an explanation). Fun facts: Ancient Greeks had their own version of lube, vibrators were created to aid women with menstrual cramps (not to treat female hysteria), the very first condom can be dated to 1560, glass dildos existed in 1800s China, and blow-up sex dolls were created in 1850s France and called "rubber women."

In our contemporary society, sex tools and toys are fairly common, especially in metropolitan areas. Most of my friends have vibrators, some have anal toys, and many use lube. What's the difference between sex toys and sex tools? Honestly, nothing. Sex educators prefer to use the term *sex tools* because that's what they actually are—they're tools to enhance your sex life. Although the term *sex toys* has been more common in the past, *toys* just doesn't seem to carry the significance or convey the benefits and pleasure these items can bring. Ultimately, though, you can use whatever term you prefer. They're the same.

Sex Tool Myths

"If you need sex toys, your sex life must not be great."

There are a lot of sex tool myths, and many of them are harmful to individuals and couples. This first one—if you use sex tools, then you must not have a great sex life or a good relationship—is a huge misconception and

[66] Angela Chen, "From Ice Age Dildos to VR, an Academic Explains the History and Future of Sex Toys," *Verge*, February 14, 2018, www.theverge.com/2018/2/14/17009834/hallie-lieberman-buzz-sex-toys-history-technology.

honestly BS. Let's look at research results[67] based on almost twelve thousand respondents. The researchers found that owning and using sex tools is associated with higher sexual satisfaction, as well as life satisfaction! The study also found the most common sex tools are vibrators, dildos, handcuffs, cock rings, and anal toys. Interestingly, the frequency of using sex tools with your partner is associated with relationship satisfaction, so make sure you don't just use your toys by yourself. Sharing is caring. Statistically[68], owning and using sex tools is way more common than you'd think; 78 percent of individuals globally have at least one sex tool!

"Strap-ons are gay."

The second myth is that sex tools are associated with a certain gender and sexual orientation. This is honestly harmful for so many reasons. Do you think only gay men have prostates?! Anal sex can be pleasurable for all men with prostates, so why does it only have to be for a specific group of people? Likewise, strap-ons are commonly used among lesbian couples, but in the last decade they've become more mainstream with heterosexual couples (e.g., the woman wears the strap-on and pleasures her man's butthole). All men can also use butt plugs and anal beads if they want to; those tools aren't just for women and gay men. It's important to reduce hostility and shame toward men who enjoy these tools because it's really OK.

67. Gert Martin Hald et al., "Do Sex Toys Make Me Satisfied? The Use of Sex Toys in Denmark, Norway, Sweden, Finland, France, and the UK," *Journal of Sex Research* (January 2024): 1–15, https://doi.org/10.1080/00224499.2024.2304575.

68. "Sex Toys Market Size, Share, Analysis, Forecast, Trend 2030," Spherical Insights, April 2023, https://www.sphericalinsights.com/reports/sex-toys-market.

"Women who use sex toys don't have sex with their partners."

Not only is this untrue, but in real life, it's quite the opposite! When women use vibrators, dildos, or anal beads in their masturbation routine, it helps them maintain their sexual well-being and build a sexual appetite. Women who use sex toys for their solo sessions and in partnered sex are going to think about sex more often, enjoy sex more, and potentially initiate sex more frequently. In short, they avoid becoming sexually dormant, which can happen to a lot of people. When I use a vibrator and cum clitorally, it makes me super horny and want to jump on my husband and ride him! I've heard similar things from many women in my life. One study[69] found that women don't usually buy sex tools that resemble their partner, and straight women often don't even buy tools that look like real penises, so they're not seeking a substitute. They're looking for a fun addition to a healthy sex life.

"Vibrators desensitize your clit."

This is a controversial topic. Many people believe this one and often engage in heated conversations with me whenever I say, "No, it doesn't." Here's the thing. There's a study[70] that found women who frequently engage in long bike rides may find reduced genital sensation. The talking point, then, is "Even bike rides desensitize the clit!" Well, if you look at the study, we're talking twenty-eight miles per day one to three times a week. That's not even comparable to women using a little vibrator for

---

69. Sarah E. Johns and Nerys Bushnell, "What Drives Sex Toy Popularity? A Morphological Examination of Vaginally-Insertable Products Sold by the World's Largest Sexual Wellness Company," *Journal of Sex Research* 61, no. 2 (February 2023): 161–168, https://doi.org/10.1080/00224499.2023.2175193.

70. Marsha K. Guess et al., "Genital Sensation and Sexual Function in Women Bicyclists and Runners: Are Your Feet Safer than Your Seat?," *Journal of Sexual Medicine* 3, no. 6 (November 2006): 1018–1027, https://doi.org/10.1111/j.1743-6109.2006.00317.x.

five to ten minutes a couple times a week. Still, it's entirely possible for someone to abuse their vibrator. People have always battled with addiction, so yeah, if you use the strongest setting on your vibrator for hours every day, every week, you could cause numbness and nerve damage. The moral of the story, though, is this: It's not the vibrator, it's how you use it. A great way to ensure your body isn't used to just one type of sensation is to have different types of vibrators that feel different from one another. Be mindful of how—and how often—you're using it.

"Men don't need sex tools to masturbate."

Technically, you can masturbate without any tools to enhance your experience, but you might not know that it can be harmful to masturbate with your dry hand with the same technique for years on end. Have you ever heard of the term *idiosyncratic masturbation*? This is where your brain and body get used to a certain type of grip, movement, and stimulation via years of masturbation, and it can cause you to be unable to orgasm through other methods, like your partner's hand, mouth, vagina, or butthole. Of course, introducing variety in your self-pleasure sessions can be beneficial. You can use lube and lotion, switch up the hand, and use sex tools such as male masturbators, sleeves, or a pocket pussy. There's no shame in the male sex toy game.

Staple Sex Tools

VIBRATORS!

Vibrators are my number one pick for women. Straight men can buy one for their partners as a gift, and single men can have one in a drawer to pleasure their dates. There are many types of vibrators, and preference is so individualized. I have many friends who love big massagers, but I'm a fan of medium- to smaller-sized vibrators. Here are a few things to consider:

Material: Most importantly, it needs to be body-safe, free of phthalates, and waterproof or water-resistant. But do you prefer soft (silicone) or hard (stainless steel) material?

Stimulation type: Do you like regular vibrations (most vibrators), a clit-sucking motion, a tongue-licking motion, or all of the above?

Size: Do you want a small, medium, or large device? Some people prefer small, dainty, and pointy, whereas others think the bigger ones are easier to hold. I used to have a very small stainless-steel vibrator in my 20s, but then I tried out the medium-sized silicone one I grew to love. Some tools are designed to grip easily, but others are poorly designed and very hard to hold. You won't know what you like until you try out a few types.

Quietness: Some vibrators are loud. Does that affect you? I've talked to some women who said they don't really care about the noise, but quietness is very important to me. I only like quiet to very quiet vibrators. This is something you'll have to investigate, research, and try out.

Design: Do you like external stimulation (clitoral vibes), internal stimulation (g-spot vibes), couple stimulation, hands-free features, or maybe all the above? For your very first vibrator, I recommend a small- to medium-sized clitoral silicone vibrator that's body-safe, waterproof, and quiet. Once you get comfortable with your first one, you can venture out to other types of vibrators and stimulation.

LUBE!

Lube is my first pick for men. I know it's not an electronic device, but it is an amazing sex tool that will significantly enhance your solo pleasure sessions and partnered sex. When I give my husband a hand job, I always try to use lube. He loves it. It's a great sensation and reduces unpleasant friction. There are many types of lube out there, so a bit of research is in order. Silicone-based lube works with most condoms, stays slick and slippery a long time, and is waterproof for shower sex or jerking off in the shower, but it stains your sheets, can cause irritation in some women's vagina, and can damage silicone toys. Water-based lube is mostly safe for the body, you can use it with condoms, and it's easy to clean up, but it dries out pretty quickly, so you need to reapply during a long jack session or sensual partnered sex. It can also create little pieces of jelly mush that many people dislike. Coconut oil–based lube is my favorite. Coconut oil is antibacterial and multipurpose, you can use it to masturbate, it's safe for vaginal and anal sex, and it's edible (so it's great for nipple play, rim jobs, blow jobs, and so on). It's also good for your skin and amazing for sensual massages. The cons are that it's not compatible with latex condoms, so make sure you get polyurethane or lambskin condoms, and some people are allergic to coconut.

EVERYTHING ELSE

Other tools I recommend are anal beads and butt plugs for people who are interested in or love butt sex, cock rings for firmer and harder cocks, male masturbators to create variety in men's masturbation routines, and remote-controlled vibrators for sexy and naughty nights out. For fun power play action and BDSM, you can try collars and leashes, handcuffs, ball gags, floggers, bondage rope, blindfolds, feather ticklers, strap-ons, and nipple clamps. Remember, you should always educate yourself in how to safely use these tools before you use them. You must also communicate with your partner in advance before bringing the tools out during sex. It can be a huge turn-off when sex tools are brought out without a proper conversation to determine if both people are into it. Imagine someone puts a ball gag on you during sex without knowing you have a deep fear of suffocation. Likewise, imagine a woman putting on a strap-on and just sliding it right into her partner's butt without previous agreement. Not OK.

How To Talk About Sex Tools

If you rarely or never talk about sex with your partner, bringing up your desire to include sex tools in the bedroom might be a bit challenging. Talking about sex is more awkward than other topics in general, and your partner might feel like they're not "enough" for you, which is untrue. Since it's a sensitive topic, you should approach it mindfully. Use my PEVIS method!

- **Start with a positive comment, such as "Sex last night was amazing, I loved spending time and being intimate with you."**
- **Explore your partner's views on the topic. For example, say, "I saw an article about fun sexy things couples can try in bed and one of the recommendations was to use a vibrator during sex. What do you think about that?"**
- **Share your vulnerability.**
- **Use I language. This could sound like "I'll be honest with you. It sounds like fun and might give me different types of orgasms. I would love for us to try."**
- **Finally, suggest a solution. For example, ask, "How about we go to a store or online and pick out one together?"**

PEVIS is an effective method that works for all sensitive sex conversations, so give it a try and let me know how it goes. It can be used to bring up topics such as sexless relationships, a desire to try new things, not feeling desired, insecurity about vaginal wetness or erectile dysfunction, and sexual feedback. Once you have a conversation about using sex tools and you're on the same page, it's time to have fun exploring and buying one (or more) tools.

Discovering online sex toy sites and in-person adult stores can be fun and exciting to do alone and with your partner, but it can also be exhausting and nerve-racking. The first time I went to a sex toy store, I was in my twenties. My friend Lori took me, and I remember feeling excited but also overwhelmed. I was pretty amazed, dazed, and slightly shocked the whole time. I remember thinking, "Wow, they have stuff for that?!" I saw everything from pig masks, huge cock-like dildos, and dick pumps to more than forty types of vibrators. Good thing Lori was able to recommend a combo pack that came with a clitoral vibrator and a g-spot vibrator.

Since then, I have been to sex stores and online sites *many* times (for . . . research). So here are my top tips for beginners:

Go to the shop or online store with an open mind and a playful attitude! Have fun looking at different tools and toys. Don't pressure yourself into buying something during your first visit. You really don't have to if you feel too overwhelmed to make a decision.

If you have something in mind that you'd like to purchase, don't hesitate to ask the staff. In most boutiques I've visited, the staff were trained to understand all the tools and what people would enjoy based on their preferences.

Be respectful to others. I once saw a group of young college students talking loudly near a woman in her 40s who was buying nipple clamps. "Eww, look! She's buying that weird nipple thing! Gross!" That's so disrespectful. Don't yuck other people's yum. Focus on your own tool-buying experience.

If you like to shop online, read the reviews and compare a few different products in the same category to see which one would suit you best. There are so many amazing sex tools out there you can enjoy!

Aftercare for Sex Tech, Toys, and Tools

Communication is key when you incorporate and use technology in your sexual relationships. Whether it's sexting, engaging in cybersex, or using sex tools, consistent communication helps couples be on the same page. After a hot sexting and cybersex session or playing with sex tools, it's important to ask your partner how they feel about it and if it was fun and pleasurable for them. Checking in afterward shows that you care and that you want the best experience to nourish both of you. If you use sex tech solo, make sure that you're mindful of your frequency and how you use it.

Chapter 9

All Fantasies Are Valid, Right?

Science tells us that these fantasies—your fantasies—are, in all likelihood, perfectly normal and healthy, and once you understand how common your sexual fantasies are, where they come from, and their deeper meaning, you will gain the ability to express your sexual desires to others.

—Dr. Justin Lehmiller, *Tell Me What You Want*

Kendall had always lied to her partner, Jason, whenever he asked about her sexual fantasies. Talking about sex in general had been a hard thing for Kendall, but after working with me individually and as a couple, she was able to gain the confidence to talk about sex-related things. For example, she learned to talk about sexual frequency desires (she wanted once a week, he wanted three times a week, but they compromised), a desire for more romance (common among women), and using sex tools in bed. Although she became more comfortable with her sexuality, she still had a big hiccup: She never wanted to talk about sexual fantasies.

"What's the point?" she asked. "I'm talking about all the things that are necessary for our sex life already. I feel like that should be enough."

I acknowledged her discomfort and explained the truth about why discussing sexual fantasies could be beneficial to her sex life.

"That's true. You have been very brave, and I admire your growth mindset. You've talked about so many things you didn't think you could when we started. If talking about sexual fantasies is a hard boundary, we can 100 percent revisit this later. I do want to let you know that by exploring and sharing your sexual fantasies, you are honoring your sexuality more fully and can contribute to really great outcomes for your sex life now and in the future."

Jason then chimed in with "Come on babe, just say it. It's just for fun! I told you mine. Fucking an alien is one of my fantasies. Like, for real. I just think it would feel so out of this world to have sex with an alien or a few of them. But I want to hear yours!"

Kendall pleaded, "Let's just table this for now, please?" I ended the session by assigning them some sexual exploration exercises.

***Trigger warning*: Content related to forced sex and suicide.** The next day, Kendall scheduled an individual session in the afternoon, which was unusual. When we started our Zoom call, she looked a bit disturbed.

"How's it going, Kendall?" I said casually. "I'm pleasantly surprised to see you before next week's call."

"I just wanted to talk about sexual fantasies or whatever with you before our next call," she said.

"Sure thing! I'm here to help you navigate this journey and answer any questions you may have," I said in a positive tone.

"I think my fantasy is really weird. I don't even know if I should say it out loud. Sometimes I think it's so sick that I fantasize about something like this. I don't ever want to mention it to Jason because I feel like he'll see me in a different light. Like seriously, I feel like it's borderline disgusting. I hate that I even think about it, but like you told me before, sometimes sexual thoughts just pop up in your head. So yeah . . . I'm down to tell you, but this is just between you and me—no Jason."

I already had a sense of what it may have been because a lot of women have variations of this fantasy and are too ashamed to talk about it. So I reassured her, "Of course! And let me tell you right now, there is nothing you can say to me about your fantasies that will make me judge you negatively. I'm here to support you and help you feel more comfortable with your sexuality."

She looked a bit more relieved. "OK, so . . . I've heard you talk about this on a podcast. I think it's called consensual nonconsent. I don't know. I fantasize about forced sex a lot—like someone is fucking me against my will and I'm fighting them off, but it's a passionate sexual encounter. The person really just craves me. They want my body, they will do everything they can to fuck me, and I always end up really liking it in the fantasy. Like it felt good, I was wet and even had an orgasm. But am I sick? Because that's like . . . rape? I feel like something's wrong with me if the thought of being forced to have sex turns me on. I really need to know if I'm normal."

News flash: Nothing was wrong with Kendall. Many women have a forced sex fantasy or rape fantasy. Researchers have studied this phenomenon[71] and found that 62 percent of women who participated in the study have had a rape fantasy. In one study[72] from 2012, researchers found that women with higher self-esteem and an openness to fantasy reported greater sexual arousals from rape-related fantasies. So, babes, nothing's wrong with you. You're just an imaginative, sexually curious human being.

After walking Kendall through the studies explaining that her fantasies were normal and experienced by many women, she gave a huge sigh of relief. "Whew, OK cool. It's great to know that I'm not alone. I

---

[71] Jenny Bivona and Joseph Critelli, "The Nature of Women's Rape Fantasies: An Analysis of Prevalence, Frequency, and Contents," *Journal of Sex Research* 46, no. 1 (February 2009): 33–45, https://doi.org/10.1080/00224490802624406.

[72] Jenny Bivona et al., "Women's Rape Fantasies: An Empirical Evaluation of the Major Explanations," *Archives of Sexual Behavior* 41, no. 5 (April 2012): 1107–1119, https://doi.org/10.1007/s10508-012-9934-6.

swear more people *need* to know this because I've lived with this shame a long time, since I was, like, nineteen. Seriously, every time I catch myself fantasizing about it, I'd feel really bad afterward. You need to teach everyone about this!"

Well, here I am! When I was planning this book, I knew in my heart that I had to have a chapter about sexual fantasies not only because it's a fun topic people are interested in but also because of what Kendall said that day. It stuck with me. How much shame do people—men, women, and nonbinary—have to live with due to their fantasies and imaginations?

You can't really choose what fantasies pop up in your head. Of course, you can cultivate the ones you want to think about: the ones that feel sexy, fun, and exciting. However, most people (myself included) have multiple fantasies that just happen—fantasies that just unintentionally pop into their mind. Many teens and young adults are confused by their unexpected fantasies, and many people don't have the resources to see a therapist or feel comfortable sharing with a professional. This is why normalizing conversations about sex, desires, and fantasies is so important.

Human imagination is *wild*! Can we all at least accept that? It's OK that we imagine things; fantasies are natural. Just look at the creativity on display in books, movies, and TV shows. People don't usually see writers and directors as sick and weird because of the art they create, but because sexual fantasies are so much more individualized, people assign personal and negative connotations to them. "She has a submissive fantasy, so she must have daddy issues." "He has an anime fantasy, so he must be a weirdo." "He has a cross-dressing fantasy, so he must be a creep." "They have a gangbang fantasy, so they must have had a terrible childhood." The world can feel like it's full of judgment and negative assumptions. Let's change that together!

Whether you fantasize about getting railed by ten hot men, getting fingered in a movie theater by your celebrity crush, or having sex with your English teacher, your fantasies are fine—and you're not weird. In fact, sexual fantasies and imagination are an important part of your sexual wellness. However, it's important to make the distinction among fantasy, obsession, and a desire to experience things in real life, which is what we will do in this chapter. We'll also take a look at relevant studies and experiments, common fantasies in the United States, ten questions to ask yourself to discover your sexual fantasy, and how to have a conversation about fantasies.

SEXUAL FANTASY 101

We all fantasize about all kinds of things. I fantasize about my dream home at the beach with two children and a Shiba Inu. My sexy husband, shirtless, is cooking lunch in our large kitchen with a beautiful marble countertop. The sun is shining, and it's a relaxing Sunday where we all sit down, have lunch together, and then play a board game. That's my fantasized home life that I very much want to make come true.

How are sexual fantasies different from other fantasies? Well, they're all about sex and usually turn you on and elicit some type of sexual arousal. Sexual fantasies are imaginary scenarios and stories, patterns of thoughts, or mental images related to sex and sexuality that create sexual arousal and may or may not involve the person that is doing the fantasizing. For example, I might fantasize about what it's like to have sex with Marvel characters. On the other hand, you can also have fantasies that don't involve you as a participant, like watching your celebrity crush masturbate. There are literally millions of possible scenarios. Just remember that a fantasy is an imaginative thought and not necessarily indicative of your real desires, related to something you're doing, or representative of something you'd ever do. If you have a fantasy that you personally find disturbing, take a few deep breaths and try not to be extremely anxious about it. Allow it to come and go. Remember, if you're not actively enacting your fantasy, it's just a thought. Seeking out sex therapy or coaching can also help you process and understand these thoughts with more clarity.

(Almost) everyone fantasizes about sex, regardless of age, gender, sexual orientation, racial background, ethnicity, country of citizenship, or socioeconomic status. Even asexual people experience sexual fantasies![73] Sexual fantasies can be an amazing tool to enhance your sex life. Often, when I talk to people who feel sexually depleted, I ask about the last time they had a sexual fantasy and what it was. They typically say, "I haven't had one in a long time" or "I just don't think about those things." Meanwhile, when I interact with people who feel like they have a satisfying sex life and ask the same question, they usually tell me about the latest thing they've been fantasizing about with positivity and a giggly tone—like they're doing something a bit mischievous.

Sexual fantasies allow people to maintain their sexuality. If you haven't thought about sex for years, then you're probably not having good sex—or having any sex at all. It's fine if you're asexual or don't have the desire to have sex, and it's quite common for people in these situations to not fantasize about sex. However, if you usually have a strong sexual appetite, fantasies help you maintain a healthy amount of sexual energy in your life. Fantasizing about sex from time to time during the day can help keep that sexual juice going. I know it works for me! Let me know if it works for you too.

Why do we have sexual fantasies? People are naturally creative and imaginative, and we're also just sexual beings. We're one of only a few species that have sex for pleasure. So it's not rocket science to conclude that we will inevitably think about random sex stuff and come up with all kinds of creative scenarios about it. But where do so-called deviant sexual fantasies come from? Well, there are five external sources: the media, modeled experience, previous sexual experiences, childhood abuse, and porn.

There is a misconception that our fantasies are always related to what happened to us in the past. Remember Kendall? She was concerned

73. *Psychology Today* Staff, "Fantasies," *Psychology Today*, www.psychologytoday.com/us/basics/fantasies.

about her fantasy and, while explaining it to me, gave the disclaimer "I don't know why this is happening to me. It's not like I was forced to have sex with someone when I was a kid." I immediately corrected her. "Oh no, actually, research[74] has found that a history of forced sex is actually unrelated to forced sex fantasies."

Another common myth is that everybody's fantasies involve their partners or spouses. Not true! Interestingly, researchers[75] found at least 42 percent of people never fantasize about their partners, and 90 percent fantasize about cheating scenarios. I think it's normal for people to have mischievous thoughts because, again, they're just a product of the imagination, not action. Is it bad that I have a sexual fantasy about someone who's not my partner? No, not at all. Having a sexual fantasy about someone doesn't mean you want to date them IRL.

Do people always want to live out their sexual fantasies? No, they don't. There's a misconception that if you fantasize about something, then it means you must want to act it out in real life, but that's far from the truth. People might want to make a couple of their fantasies come true, but that's not the case for all fantasies. Think of it this way: There's feasible fantasy, probable fantasy, and just-a-fantasy. Feasible fantasies are those that we believe are doable and unchallenging to try if we have the desire and opportunity. Probable fantasies are more challenging and harder to do in real life, but if we have the desire and opportunity, we may wait for the suitable time and the right people. By contrast, a just-a-fantasy is a type of sexual fantasies we know is impossible or that we'd never want to do in real life. For me, a feasible fantasy is getting fingered in a movie theater, a probable fantasy is a passionate and fun foursome at Burning Man, and a just-a-fantasy is getting abducted by aliens and forced to have sex with them on an alien ship.

---

74. Christian C. Joyal et al., "What Exactly Is an Unusual Sexual Fantasy?," *Journal of Sexual Medicine* 12, no. 2 (February 2015): 328–340, https://doi.org/10.1111/jsm.12734.
75. Brett Kahr, *Who's Been Sleeping in Your Head: The Secret World of Sexual Fantasies* (Basic Books, 2009).

When should we be cautious about unusual fantasies and take them more seriously? Notably, if you start having a desire to make illegal fantasies come true, such as engaging in rape in real life or having sex with an animal. When you're in the desire stage, it means you *want* to make your fantasies real, and that's not OK when they involve illegal activities. You need to find remedies for these desires by understanding them and seeking treatment before you act on them. This is where seeing a sex therapist, psychologist, or even psychiatrist can be crucial. When certain sexual fantasies become behaviors, they can be problematic and detrimental. Still, it's very important not to shame someone who shares these desires with you because it might make them even more ashamed of themselves and backfire in a form of self-harm or harming others. The best thing to do in this scenario is to recommend that person see a professional.

Top Five Sexual Fantasies in the United States

Women are almost always treated as if they are less sexual than men—or that they shouldn't have more sexual desire than men—which often leads to shame and misunderstanding. What really helped me overcome this was reading erotica from women's perspectives because it showed me that I'm not alone. Some of my favorite examples include *My Secret Garden*, *Forbidden Flowers*, *Beyond My Control*, and *Women on Top* by the iconic Nancy Friday. They all deal with women's sexual fantasies, and the focus is on women maintaining control of their own sexual desires and outcomes.

Another critically acclaimed book about sexual fantasies is *Tell Me What You Want* by Justin Lehmiller. I love this book and highly recommend it because it's both educational and accessible. It helped me feel more comfortable with my and other people's sexual fantasies. In the book, Lehmiller ranked Americans' favorite sexual fantasies, which he determined from conversations with more than four thousand people. The most popular fantasy doesn't surprise me at all. I've heard this fantasy from countless people, and it's consistently one of the most popular categories on porn sites: *threesomes*! To be more specific, it's group sex or multi-partnered sex.

Here's how the rest of the top five played out:

1. **Threesomes (group sex with more than one partner or multipartnered sex)**
2. **Power and control (e.g., rough sex, forced sex, BDSM)**
3. **Novelty, adventure, and variety (e.g., sex in unconventional places, unexpected and thrilling sexual encounters, food play, sex tools, sex tech, pegging)**
4. **Forbidden sex (e.g., watching other people have sex, having sex while people watch, engaging in incest, engaging in bestiality, having sex with "adult babies" and furries)**
5. **Passion, romance, and intimacy (e.g., being wanted and desired by someone)**

What do you think? Any of those fantasies pique your interest? I know that all this can feel a little overwhelming, so in the next section, I will help you navigate and find out what sexual fantasies you might be into that are just waiting for you to mindfully explore.

Seven Categories of Sexual Fantasy

Sexual Identity: This can include fantasies related to same-sex sexual encounters, cross-dressing, gender swapping, gender fluidity, sex with a trans person, and imagining yourself as queer or trans.

Multiple Partners and Nonmonogamy: This can include fantasies related to threesomes, foursomes, group sex, orgies, gang bangs, reverse gang bangs, swinging, cuckolding, polyamory, polygamy, polyandry, sex parties, circle jerks, double penetration, and airtight fantasies (e.g., when all the holes filled).

Power and Control: This can include fantasies related to bondage, discipline, domination and submission, sadism, masochism, power play, impact play, spanking, slapping, flogging, punishment, electrostimulation, forced sex scenarios, gagging, choking, torture, chastity, collars, leashes, puppy play, pony play, adult babies, breast bondage, cock whipping, ball crushing, knife play, and slave and master scenarios.

Fun Variety and Novelty: This can include fantasies related to outdoor sex, surprised sex, sex games, naked painting, cosplay, role play, blindfolds, handcuffs, sex in the shower, sex in the pool, sex with a stranger, sex with a celebrity, sex with a teacher, temperature play, sex with aliens, sex in weird places, tickling, strip teases, lingerie, and food play.

Illegal or Immoral: This can include fantasies related to rape, forced sex, incest, sex with animals, sex with underage people, sex with corpses, sex with people in a coma, sex to spread STDs, groping people in crowded places, touching people sexually in their sleep, and cannibalism. If you're experiencing this kind of fantasy, the first step is to remove shame from it and remember that just because you have these thoughts doesn't mean you want to act them out. However, if it's distressing you or if you start to feel an urge to act, you should seek professional help and talk to a therapist as soon as possible.

Romance and Passion: This can include fantasies related to passionate sex with your partner, getting swept away, receiving a love letter, sensual massage, tantric sex, sexual meditation, pussy worship, cock worship, naked cuddling, sex with an ex, eye gazing, making out, French kissing, body kissing, romantic words, and sex on a bed full of rose petals.

Sexual Acts and Positions: This can include fantasies related to oral sex, receiving a happy ending, anal sex, vaginal penetration, fingering, rimming, face-sitting, creampies, deep throating, fisting, bukkake, cheating, mutual masturbation, having sex while other people watch, watching people have sex, fetishes, period sex, sex with poop, water sports, teabagging, squirting, snowballling, cake farts, blow jobs, hand jobs, clit rubbing, and clit sucking.

Five Questions to Ask Yourself to Discover Your Sexual Fantasy

1. **What are some sexual things that you're curious about but wouldn't ever want to do in real life?**
2. **If you can do whatever you want, with no consequences, what sexual things might you do?**
3. **Fantasies are not real life, so if you have an assignment to create the wildest and sexiest porn video, what would you include?**
4. **Do you think you're a powerful person? Do you like thinking about enacting that power during sex in a reasonable or taboo way? Or do you prefer thinking about yielding and being submissive?**
5. **What are some of your favorite settings (e.g., mountains, theme parks, movies)? If you insert a sexual act into that setting, what does it look like?**

After answering these questions, you'll be able to discover quite a few sexual fantasies for yourself. Now, in order to use that information to enhance your sexual power, you must use it mindfully. If you find yourself obsessing over your fantasies, pull back, do breathwork and meditation, and remind yourself that there's no shame in the therapy game. Overall, fantasizing about sexual things can be healthy and beneficial for your sexual wellness.

How to Have a Conversation About Sexual Fantasies

The short answer is with an open mind and curiosity! The more comprehensive answer is that you need to find a relaxing time to discuss sexual fantasies, whether it's with your partner or a friend, hanging out on the couch, on a road trip, taking a walk on the beach, during a wine night, on a sexy date night, or the like. Sharing your fantasies can feel extremely empowering and liberating because you're verbalizing sexual thoughts that are very personal to you. Again, many times, these fantasies are taboo, so communicating them out loud can serve our rebellious souls—but don't push yourself too hard to share your deepest fantasies with a new partner if your gut feeling tells you to wait. There should be a safe space in all relationships and a healthy amount of trust between you before you share your fantasies. Know that you're not obligated to share anything you're not ready to; when you want to share your fantasies, it should come from an empowering place rather than fear or people-pleasing behavior. It's also completely OK if you want to keep your fantasies near and dear to yourself without sharing them with anyone else.

If you're the one inquiring, don't just ask, "What's your sexual fantasy?" Give more context about why you're interested and share that you won't judge them. For example, say, "I've been reading Dr. Tara's book, and she discusses sexual fantasies and how talking about them can bring couples closer together. So I've been thinking about mine and I'm curious what yours are. Would you like to share some of your sexual fantasies? No judgment here, just curiosity and an open mind!" As you can see, this is so much more comfortable and validating than blurting out "What is your sexual fantasy?"

When someone shares their sexual fantasies with you, especially the more taboo ones, it means that they really trust you. They trust that you won't judge them or think they're a bad person for having those thoughts. This brings me to a very important tip about engaging in a conversation about sexual fantasies: Try to engage in active and nonjudgmental listening as much as possible. Everyone is entitled to their own opinion. You may disagree with, dislike, or even feel disgust with someone's sexual fantasy, but it's best not to outwardly express negative judgment because that will break trust and ruin the relationship in small and big ways. Recognize that it takes a lot of courage to share your deepest, darkest sexual fantasies. Most people have them, even if they're not talking about them.

When Fantasies Come True (the Good, the Bad, and the Ugly)

"Ugh, the first time we had a threesome was terrible. I didn't cum. My boyfriend was looking at our third the whole time. He just focused on pounding, and I was, like, there as an accessory. We made eye contact maybe once or twice. I didn't want to be a party pooper, so I pretended to enjoy all of it, but I was legit waiting for it to end." The funny (and shitty) thing about this experience is that it's a pretty common account of people's first time having a threesome. I've never heard anyone say that the first threesome they had was the best sex of their life. Literally no one has told me that, and I know a lot of people who have had threesomes. That's the thing about sexual fantasies: A lot of them seem great in your mind, but they're not that great in person. We're imaginative creatures, and our minds can invent so many things beyond the actual things we can do and accomplish during our lifetimes.

Having in a threesome (or group sex) is the most popular sexual fantasy in the United States, but how many people actually have one in real life? Out of those people, how many enjoyed it? Like, *really* enjoyed it? Interestingly, research[76] found that most people who have had threesomes

---

76. Hannah Morris et al., "Three's a Crowd or Bonus?: College Students' Threesome Experiences," *Journal of Positive Sexuality* 2, no. 3 (October 2016): 62–76, https://doi.org/10.51681/1.234.

only did it once and didn't try it again. (Granted, the participants in that study were college students, so we don't necessarily know if they decided to try it again when they got older.) When asked about the consequences of that sexual experience, most couples said it had no effect on their relationship, 17 percent said it brought them closer together, 14 percent said it put a strain on the relationship, and 7 percent said it ended the relationship. Having a threesome can be a great time that brings a lot of fun and pleasure to your sex life when done with care, consent, and a lot of communication. But just like many other sexual fantasies, people tend to act it out only once to see what it's like. A much smaller percentage of people decide to engage in them regularly in real life.

What if this is only one partner's fantasy and the other is not OK with it? It's all good! You can always try role-play. Role-play allows people to "live" in a fantasy world for a limited time. A friend once acted like a creepy male gynecologist (remember, it's just role-play; he's actually an engineer in real life) to have fantasy sex with his girlfriend who acted as his patient ready to be taken advantage of. Acting out a fantasy can be a bonding activity that offers excitement and novelty for long-term couples. It can be an amazing, liberating, and exciting feeling to share with your partner. In addition to more realistic fantasies, my partner and I also talk about other fantasies that we don't ever want to do in real life. They're either impossible or immoral, but we still share with each other because we trust that our relationship is a judgment-free zone. If you don't want to partake in your partner's fantasy, it's good to have a conversation about why it's a turn-off for you and then find a compromise on what is acceptable and hot for your relationship. For instance, a client wanted to try a threesome with her husband, but he really didn't want to try, so they compromised by watching porn together instead.

Lastly, I won't do this chapter justice if I don't also discuss the "ugly." I'm not oblivious. I know the world of sexuality isn't all kittens and rainbows. I know there are sick people out there who commit hideous sex crimes based on their sexual fantasies. These actions are completely unacceptable, and there must be proper consequences for those who engage in them. Nonconsensual sex, rape, child molestation, and other forms of illegal sexual activities cause detrimental harm to the victims and the people around them, and they should never be taken lightly. The people committing these crimes usually lack empathy, like to manipulate others, and get off on exploiting them. Research[77] found that psychopathy is the significant link between having deviant sexual fantasies and acting them out in real life. I should note, though, that it's not that common. Sexual fantasies, like most things in life, have good and bad aspects. As responsible sex-positive people, we can normalize talking about them so we can explore the good and prevent the bad.

Aftercare for Acting Out a Sexual Fantasy

Many people have acted out their sexual fantasies only to find that their fantasies didn't turn out the way they wanted to or had hoped for. That's why it's essential to debrief after the act of making your fantasy come true. Open-ended questions like "How was it, baby?" "What did you think about that?" and "Would you try that again?" can help facilitate a more open-minded and empathetic conversation. Remember not to take feedback too personally and use it as a baseline for the future, whether you're trying out the same fantasy again or moving on to the next. For instance, after going to our first sex party together, I asked my partner how it was for him, what he would have done differently, what parts he enjoyed the most, if there were anything else I could have done to improve

77. Kevin M. Williams et al., "Inferring Sexually Deviant Behavior from Corresponding Fantasies: The Role of Personality and Pornography Consumption," *Criminal Justice and Behavior* 36, no. 2 (December 2008): 198–222, https://doi.org/10.1177/0093854808327277

the experience, and what he found most surprising about the whole thing. This was an insightful and fun conversation to have. We ended up laughing about a bunch of different things that happened while we ate ramen at home at 3 a.m. Life can be magical when you feel comfortable sharing your fantasies without a fear of judgment.

Chapter 10

Porn Is Not Your Enemy: How to Use Porn to Enhance Your Sex Life

Ethical porn is a partnership. A sexy, slippery, hot, heavy, and dirty partnership between people who love to fuck in front of cameras and people who love to watch them do it.

—David Ley, *Ethical Porn for Dicks*

Marcus started watching porn and masturbating when he was fourteen years old. For the next ten years, he consumed porn almost every day, sometimes multiple times a day, not knowing that his porn habits would become a big issue later in life. In his mid-twenties, he realized that he had become dependent on porn to gain pleasure, get an erection, and orgasm. This realization caused an enormous amount of dating and sexual anxiety. He was extremely nervous whenever he was on a date, especially when it was time to escalate to the passionate moment. He couldn't do it. He'd panic, make an excuse to go home, and never talk to that woman again. Other times, he would be able to stay focused and have a nice make-out session with his date, but when it came to getting hard, his erection was unreliable. Sometimes he would be hard for a few minutes; other times he couldn't get hard at all. This situation affected relationships with more than a dozen women over three years.

He came to me in his late twenties, after he had been dating Emily for three months. They hadn't had sex yet, but the thought of it made him anxious enough to look for solutions. That's when he stumbled on my work.

"Dr. Tara! I listened to your podcast about your friend named Matt and his journey to overcome porn dependency and anxiety," said Marcus in an excitable but nervous tone. "I realized that's probably what I have. I haven't been able to get hard with a partner for many years now, and I honestly don't know what to do at this point. I'm dating someone I really like, but we haven't had sex." The friend Marcus had mentioned bravely shared on my podcast that he'd been excessively watching porn since his early teen years, which had negatively affected him in terms of building intimacy with a woman in real life. He was experiencing so much sexual anxiety that he didn't have his first sexual experience until he was twenty-seven years old.

I responded, "I'm glad you listened to that episode, so you know you're not alone. Feeling lonely and ashamed regarding porn use can worsen the situation. About eleven percent of men[78] believe they're addicted to porn. In fact, they've just not been taught to use it mindfully. We will need to do a whole reset and reboot. Is that OK? Are you open to an intervention?"

Marcus immediately jumped in with, "Honestly, at this point, I'll do anything. I was thinking maybe I'd just take Viagra for the rest of my life, but I really don't want to rely on a drug for sex—especially when I'm still in my twenties."

---

78. Joshua B. Grubbs et al., "Self-Reported Addiction to Pornography in a Nationally Representative Sample: The Roles of Use Habits, Religiousness, and Moral Incongruence," *Journal of Behavioral Addictions* 8, no. 1 (January 2019): 88–93, https://doi.org/10.1556/2006.7.2018.134.

"I'll be honest with you," I calmly assured him. "The intervention will take time and won't be as fast as taking a pill, but it's totally worth it considering long-term sexual fulfillment."

"OK," he said with optimism. "I'm ready for it. I'm all in. Whatever it takes."

After our first session, we met twice a week for a month so he could report his progress and discuss his journey. His intervention involved porn fasting (not watching porn for a month, not because porn is evil but to reset his habitual behavior), mindfully masturbating solely from memory once or twice a week while not rushing to orgasm (edging a few times every solo session), using different sex tools during these sessions (e.g., pocket pussy, masturbator, sleeves) to experience a variety of sensations, using lube while masturbating, engaging in sexual meditation for five minutes every day, and journaling for five minutes every day. After one month, Marcus's sexual anxiety levels dropped significantly. (If he was at a 10 out of 10 before, he dropped to a 5 out of 10.) He learned how to control his anxiety and was able to get and maintain an erection when he and Emily had sex for the first time.

In our final session, he popped on Zoom with a smile on his face, and I immediately said, "How was the sex?"

Marcus described, "Oh, sex with Emily was amazing. It was even better than I had imagined. I knew we were compatible in life, but we're also compatible in bed. We connected so well, and she was just so sexy in bed. I really appreciate all your help. Thanks, doc!" It's moments like this that fuel me to continue doing what I do best: helping people become comfortable with their sexual selves and achieve their sexual goals.

A popular porn site with more than three million videos recently shared that it gets more than five *billion*[79] visits per month. Does that number shock you? As a sex educator, it still shocks me. That's about

79. Statista Research Department, "OnlyFans—Statistics & Facts." Statista, July 2, 2024, www.statista.com/topics/10083/onlyfans/.

166 million visits per day and almost 7 million visits every hour! It's honestly staggering, especially when people use it without any education about it. Meanwhile, over the last decade, a group of scholars and therapists have warned people that porn viewing is bad—that watching porn is a recipe for disastrous relationship development.

Ultimately, there are three camps of people: those who watch too much porn, those who are against porn, and those who use porn mindfully and seek out high-quality porn. How do you watch porn? Some studies show that porn is great for couples when used correctly[80]. It can help couples get out of a routine, spice up their sex lives, and find new positions and sexual appetite for new sexual acts.

Let me stress: Porn is not your enemy. It has a bad reputation because so much of it hasn't focused on women's pleasure. Women are often objectified in porn, and sometimes women's sexual health and desires are ignored completely. I've seen a porn clip where a hot guy enters a room, approaches a woman, lifts her skirt, and inserts his dick while she moans loudly (ostensibly indicating immense pleasure). WTF? That's not how pleasure works for us!

In this chapter, I will share ways to use tools to your advantage so you can become a better lover and experience more fun, passion, and pleasure in your solo and partnered sex. My hope is that I can help you better understand mindful porn consumption and that not all porn is created the same—or that it produces the same effect in all viewers. We'll also take a look at the benefits and potential dangers as documented by research. Overall, the goal is to help people move from a place of shame regarding porn use to a place of empowerment that stems from knowing how to use it.

---

80. Nicholas P. Newstrom and Steven M. Harris, "Pornography and Couples: What Does the Research Tell Us?," *Contemporary Family Therapy* 38, no. 4 (December 2016): https://www.researchgate.net/publication/307620661_Pornography_and_Couples_What_Does_the_Research_Tell_Us.

MINDFUL VERSUS MINDLESS PORN CONSUMPTION

Porn itself isn't a weapon against humanity. How people use it, though, can make it bad. If I own and have access to a bunch of kitchen knives, I'm not necessarily going to run out of my house with them and stab a bunch of people. Realistically, I'm just going to use them to cut up ingredients, prepare meals, and nourish my body. The same thing is true with porn. Just because I have access to millions of porn videos doesn't mean I'll necessarily become a porn addict. Many people use porn as a tool to learn and explore new things in mindful ways. Most people don't spend hours every day watching porn, but the act of porn viewing has, over the last decade, been identified and talked about as "shameful behavior"—regardless of the type of porn and how people use it.

I think that narrative causes so much unnecessary anxiety in our society. Instead, we should focus on educating people. Like David Ley said in his book[81], "Belief in porn addiction is really about shame. . . . If you watch porn these days and worry about it, it's hard not to end up worried that you're a porn addict. . . . [And] believing that you're a porn addict actually makes things worse. Research has found that people who believe they're porn addicts experience more distress, more worry, more fear, and more pain. . . . The label . . . has become a form of shame and fear toward our desires for sex."

Ultimately, you don't have to abuse porn and have it negatively affect your life. You can use it mindfully, carefully, and with more intention to your advantage. Mindful porn consumption is using porn intentionally for a purpose; being aware of the frequency, duration, and type of porn you're watching; and regulating your behavior so you don't become dependent on it in order to experience pleasure. For example, I may watch porn about once a week when I masturbate. (Other times, I

---

81. David J. Ley, *Ethical Porn for Dicks: A Man's Guide to Responsible Viewing Pleasure* (Stone Bridge Press, 2016).

use my imagination or listen to audio porn.) Because I use it relatively infrequently, it doesn't have a negative impact on my sex life. I still love getting it on with my husband in sensual vanilla ways and kinky animalistic ways. I'm not desensitized by porn and can have pleasure and cum whenever I want. I use porn responsibly during my solo pleasure time to bring novelty to it. My husband and I also occasionally watch porn together (maybe once a month) as one of many tools for excitement and novelty. It's fabulous!

By contrast, mindless porn consumption is when people form a habit or routine of watching porn every time they masturbate, not being aware of how long and how often they watch it, not regulating what type of porn they watch, and essentially becoming dependent on porn for pleasure and orgasms. When you use porn compulsively and mindlessly for a long period of time (e.g., more than five hours per week over six weeks)[82], it's going to have an obvious negative impact on your life. You'll likely develop anxiety, erectile dysfunction, or an inability to orgasm.

I hope you recognize that you have the power to use porn however you'd like, so use it to amplify—not destroy—your sex life!

TYPES OF PORN (AND USING IT TO YOUR ADVANTAGE)

Video Porn

Mainstream porn is currently the most popular type of video porn because it's easily accessible and mostly free. Note, though, that it's mainly made for male audiences with actors who may not get paid or treated ethically, and many videos have limited or unrealistic portrayals of women's desire and pleasure. I'm not saying all mainstream porn is bad. There are hundreds if not thousands of categories and subcategories. You can find

82. Beth Levine, "Does Using Porn Lead to Erectile Dysfunction?," *EverydayHealth.com*, July 22, 2020, www.everydayhealth.com/erectile-dysfunction/pornography-habit-is-linked-to-erectile-dysfunction-research-suggests/.

everything from POV to gang bangs to creampies on large popular porn sites. According to Pornhub, the top ten searched-for terms in the world were *hentai, milf, lesbian, Japanese, Pinay, anal, Asian, Latina, big ass,* and *stepmom*. You can kind of get a feel for where our society is based on the top porn searches. The most popular search term in the world—by a wide margin—was *hentai,* anime porn!

A good way to use mainstream porn to your advantage is exploration (getting new ideas to try in real life or to fantasize) and education (learning new terms and moves). I would not recommend watching mainstream hardcore porn to masturbate every time because I've seen the negative ramifications of it on a lot of people (e.g., sexual anxiety, an inability to have sex with a partner in real life, and unrealistic expectations of what sex in real life should be like).

Ethical porn is the type of porn I fully support because, let's be real, porn is never going away, so if people are going to consume porn no matter what, this is the type that's best for everyone involved. Research[84] has identified aspects of porn that support healthy sexual development: It's ethically produced (i.e., it's legal and everyone gets paid fairly and treated respectfully); it shows safe sex; it focuses on pleasure for everyone involved; it shows consent communication; it includes people of different races, genders, and body types; and it shows a variety of sexual practices. Sites like CHEEX, Lust Cinema, and Make Love Not Porn showcase videos that meet these criteria. Ethical porn is sexy, hot, and features real pleasure, so I prefer this type of video if I want to watch something while masturbating. They also usually have more creative plots and depict a lot more passion and emotion. The casting is typically great, so the chemistry between performers just feels a lot more real, which makes me feel way hornier than some random internet porn that

84. Alan McKee et al., "The criteria to identify pornography that can support healthy sexual development for young adults: Results of an international Delphi Panel," *International Journal of Sexual Health* 35, no. 1 (January 2023): 1–12, https://doi.org/10.1080/19317611.2022.2161030.

has poor casting and people are just doing rough penetration without emotion or chemistry (boring!).

Creator porn is homemade, amateur, and self-produced. Basically, it's porn created by the people who are featured in them. People can share videos directly to porn sites, adult creator sites, or their own subscription platforms. This phenomenon is called the democratization of porn because anyone from anywhere with an idea, a camera, a computer, and the internet can make money by making and selling porn videos directly to viewers without traditional gatekeepers (e.g., a production company, cast, director, producer).

This movement started a long time ago but has really exploded with the rise of high-speed internet and the creator economy. There are many online sites that empower adult content creators to produce their own explicit content and get paid directly from subscribers (while the sites take a certain percentage). OnlyFans has more than two million creators and over two hundred million registered users.[85] Shockingly, according to a *Business Insider* article that interviewed eight creators on OnlyFans, these creators reportedly make somewhere from $143,000 to $5.4 million annually.[86] As a curious sex scholar, I looked into research related to this phenomenon and found some interesting tidbits. You may think most users are lonely single men, but research[87] suggests otherwise: Users are predominantly married white males. They may be looking for education, exploration, and stress relief, or they may be lonely in their marriage and seeking online companionship. Another study[88] found that OnlyFans users

---

85. Statista Research Department, "OnlyFans - Statistics & Facts."
86. Marta Biino, "How Much Money OnlyFans Creators Make," *Business Insider*, May 9, 2024, www.businessinsider.com/how-much-money-onlyfans-creators-make-real-examples-2023-1?op=1.
87. Stacey Diane Litam et al., "Sexual Attitudes and Characteristics of OnlyFans Users," *Archives of Sexual Behavior* 51, no. 6 (July 2022): 3093–3103, https://doi.org/10.1007/s10508-022-02329-0.
88. Marie Lippmann et al., "Learning on OnlyFans: User Perspectives on Knowledge and Skills Acquired on the Platform," *Sexuality & Culture* 27, no. 4 (January 2023): 1203–1223, https://doi.org/10.1007/s12119-022-10060-0.

reported a positive impact on their sex lives. Just like other categories of porn, using creator porn mindfully and carefully is the best approach.

Did you know that you can watch people have different kinds of sex for real and learn about their moves and techniques? Sounds great, right? This is called educational or instructional porn. If you search for this term, you'll find thousands of videos about squirting techniques, BDSM, different sex positions, fingering, sensual massage, how to have a threesome, and temperature play, just to name a few. Just like everything else, it's important to evaluate these videos for quality and to identify the more informed ones. There are plenty of great instructional porn videos that are well made and thoughtful, but there are also countless shitty ones that were made as a cash grab and nothing else. Here are a few tips to spot the good ones:

- **The instructor introduces themselves, their credibility, and why they want to do this video.**
- **They go step-by-step as they explain how to do that sexual act.**
- **If it involves other actor(s), they ask for consent and feedback on the scene.**
- **Everyone looks like they're excited to be there to teach you, and no one looks like they're forced to be there (unless it's about consensual nonconsent).**
- **The website has comments and reviews, which is a great way to gauge the quality.**

Audio Porn/Erotica/Erotic Content

Story porn is like a porn audiobook that can span multiple genres (e.g., passionate hookups, a threesome, sex with your ex, BDSM fantasy). The stories are well written, vividly told, and will make your legs shake and your heart beat faster. Although the stories are completely fictional, I sometimes become so engrossed that I feel like I have become the narrator. It's fascinating how much, in the absence of visual stimulations from video porn, your mind can tune into the audio and create intimate visuals for you. The horniness I feel from listening to these stories sometimes overrides the stimulation I get from old-school video porn.

Think about how much we appreciate music and lyrics and how seamlessly it has been embedded into our lives. Most people listen to music and get emotional as a result. Audio can have an intensely emotional effect on us. Now shift your perspective. If you're open to audio porn (I use the app Quinn, which is reasonably priced and has hundreds of recordings), it can enhance your sexual imagination, increase your sexual desires, and prompt you to try new things. Story porn gives me an opportunity to fantasize by listening and imagining, which is also a helpful switch from relying on visuals. We already spend too much time looking at screens, so I recommend mixing audio porn into your masturbation routine and your partnered explorations.

I didn't know real sex audio porn existed until recently, but now I think it's such a cool way to get audibly stimulated. This one is literally self-explanatory—it's listening to people have live sex. That can be someone masturbating and letting us in on the action, a couple having sex and sharing the audio with their online community, or a group enjoying an orgy or gang bang while doing a live audio broadcast. This is another fun way to explore eroticism alone or with your partner. If you have sex with your partner while listening to another couple have sex, it almost feels like swinging but without the nonmonogamy part, which makes it much more accessible to monogamous couples who want to explore something kinky!

ASMR (Autonomous Sensory Meridian Response) is a category of audio porn that really blew up in the last ten years. It became incredibly popular during the COVID-19 pandemic, when everyone was bored and anxious at home trying to find new ways to blissfully stimulate themselves out of boredom. Since then, I've seen more and more people get into ASMR for relaxation and recreational purposes. Just like other types of porn, there are many genres. One of the most popular styles of sex ASMR is when the creator acts like they're having sex with the listener. I recently came across an ASMR creator acting like she's giving a man a blow job (with all the appropriate sounds and moaning). I don't have a dick but, damn, it was so sexy, I felt like I got a boner! Another cool example I found was from a male creator who acts like he's the listener's dominant lover in bed telling her what to do and when she can cum. It's all very hot and personal. Many ASMR audios are more soothing and sensual because they are created to guide relaxing masturbation.

Erotica/Erotic Literature

"Why watch porn when you can read it?" said every kinky book lover who prefers their mind to be teased and stimulated to feel sexually aroused. The word *erotica* has its roots in Eros, the Greek god of love and passion, and I believe most good erotica really captures that word. Although the history of sexy written words can be dated back thousands of years, its popularity has been declining recently with the rise of internet porn. However, my friends at Aurore (readaurore.com) have brought back the art of writing, sharing, and reading erotica. As the site boldly claims, "Mainstream porn is not for us." On this site, you can write and share your sex stories as well as read other people's sexy stories.

There are also lots of published erotic books in various genres. From modern twisted romance novels with graphic erotic content (e.g., *Wicked Ties* by Shayla Black) to personal and kinky stories (e.g., *My Secret Garden* by Nancy Friday) to erotic BDSM novels (e.g., Anne Rice's *The Sleeping Beauty Quartet*), there are hundreds of thousands of erotica books out there for you to explore. If you don't usually like to read, I'd still give it a try as a reset for your media-strained brain—or you can listen to them as audiobooks. I was listening to "Priest" by Sierra Simone in the car the other day as I was driving home from an acupuncture appointment, and damn, it made me so horny. Seriously, try it; your sexuality will thank you.

Pornographic Photos

Sexy pictures and photos have been around for ages. Even before the invention of the camera, people were painting and sketching naked models and then selling or giving their art pieces to collectors. In the modern world, it's easy to correlate watching video porn with jerking off, but before people (mostly men) started jerking off to internet porn, previous generations were masturbating to photos in sexy magazines like *Playboy* and *Penthouse*. Nowadays, there are explicit photos everywhere online and there are so many different types of photos that it can be hard to know where to look. Whatever you're into, though, know that looking at a sexy photo, a photo of people having sex, or a photo of someone doing a sexual act while masturbating isn't shameful. You're just appreciating the eroticism.

It's healthy to sometimes use photos to invoke sexual excitement, rather than relying on video porn all the time, but I must note that this is a different behavior than being addicted to social media and following a ton of sexy Instagram models. Social media addiction is a whole different issue that should be looked into by working with a therapist or a life coach. It's not a habit that will help anyone live a more fulfilling life.

BENEFITS AND DANGERS OF PORN

Research[89] found that one of the main reasons why people watch porn is to enhance their sexual performance. Therefore, sex education is the first benefit of porn. Yes, I said it. Of course, porn is not for kids (if that didn't

---

89. Vlad Burtăverde et al., "Why Do People Watch Porn? An Evolutionary Perspective on the Reasons for Pornography Consumption," *Evolutionary Psychology* 19, no. 2 (April 2021): https://doi.org/10.1177/14747049211028798.

go without saying), but it can be helpful for adults who want to learn. Even as a university professor who teaches about sexuality, I sometimes turn to porn to further my own education. The question isn't "Can you learn from porn?" but "Which kind of porn can you learn from?" Before I was able to squirt, I watched a few instructional porn videos to learn about the elements of squirting orgasms and how to guide my partner to help me get there.

Many clients have also told me how helpful it was when I recommended educational porn to them. I had been coaching a couple who were together for eight years and really wanted to spice things up by trying new and kinky positions. Watching educational porn together was a turn-on and made it easier for them to get into those kinky positions. I also coached a single guy who wanted to learn different types of foreplay and upgrade his sex skills after a long-term relationship. I showed him educational porn videos about "foreplay tips" and "how to touch a woman," which boosted his sexual confidence. A few months later, he told me he was dating someone and the educational porn videos really helped him gain confidence and assertiveness in the bedroom. Remember: Not all porn videos are great sex education, so it's important to be aware and carefully evaluate the sources.

A lot of people say they watch porn as a stress relief.[90] The ability to tune out of reality and tune into sexual excitement serves as an effective stress reduction strategy for adults. With the right mindset and careful usage of porn, I can see how it's beneficial in helping people reduce stress, improve mood, and maintain good mental and emotional health.[91] Another potential benefit of porn is relationship enhancement. I know it sounds counterintuitive: How does watching other people have sex improve your own sex life? Well, it's more about discovering new things with your partner and having that shared (taboo) experience. If watch-

90. Arash Emamzadeh, "New Research: 8 Common Reasons People Use Porn," *Psychology Today*, May 9, 2021, www.psychologytoday.com/us/blog/finding-new-home/202105/new-research-8-common-reasons-people-use-porn.
91. Burtăverde et al., "Why Do People Watch Porn?."

ing porn makes you feel a little guilty, how liberating is it to be able to watch and enjoy it with your partner? I know it's not everybody's cup of tea, but I think it's a great way to spice things up in the bedroom from time to time. The ability to engage in this activity in a vulnerable way without judgment can significantly enhance closeness and emotional intimacy within a relationship. If you're single, porn can also help you explore your sexual fantasies and develop a healthy sexual imagination. At the end of the day, beneficial porn consumption is definitely possible, depending on the type of porn you use and how you use it. The power is in your hands.

Then there's porn addiction—a buzzword that has been flying around for the last fifteen years. People all around the world feel like they have porn addiction, as evidenced by the subreddit r/PornAddiction, which has more than fifty-nine thousand members actively sharing their stories and experiences. Although porn addiction is *not* diagnosable, Problematic Online Porn Use (POPU)[92] is the most prevalent subtype of hypersexual disorder, which is an intense focus on sexual urges, fantasies, and uncontrollable behaviors that include excessive masturbation and porn consumption. When it comes to porn, there are many types of excessive users:

- **A brain cookie user loves the hits of feel-good hormones and can't control their urges.**
- **A depressive user experiences depression and uses porn to feel more "balanced."**
- **An escapist uses porn to escape from other situations they have going on in their lives.**
- **A hidden user is unsatisfied with their current relationship and uses porn to avoid having sexual interactions with their partner.**

---

92. Rubén de Alarcón, Javier I. de la Iglesia, Nerea M. Casado, and Angel L. Montejo, "Online Porn Addiction: What We Know and What We Don't—A Systematic Review," *Journal of Clinical Medicine* 8, no. 1 (January 2019): 91, https://doi.org/10.3390/jcm8010091.

Whatever someone's reason for excessive porn use may be, they can definitely overcome it. I've heard many stories of people overcoming excessive porn use, and it's not through shame—it's by creating a fulfilling life off the internet. Once that happens, porn doesn't have a negative influence on their life; they're able to occasionally view porn and reap its benefits.

Desensitization effect is another danger that usually comes from excessive porn viewing. It happens when watching "regular" porn becomes boring, so you consistently increase the excitement and novelty by watching more and more hardcore and "unusual" porn. These users also exhibit diminished desire to have sex with their partner—but not a diminished desire to watch porn and masturbate.[93] It's unfortunately true that porn has the power to destroy romantic relationships if used mindlessly. Within heterosexual relationships, when a male partner reports increased porn use, the female partner often reports loss of emotional and psychological trust in the relationship.[94] Ultimately, there's a distinct correlation between porn consumption and probability of divorce.[95] Porn doesn't necessarily cause relationship problems, but people who are already dissatisfied with their relationship could end up relying on porn to gain sexual satisfaction, which exacerbates the strain on the relationship and can result in breakups and divorces. Therefore, it's important to be mindful when you watch porn so it doesn't impact your daily life and the well-being of your relationships. And if you have relationship issues, don't ignore them; communicate and work on the issues together.

---

93. Vaughn R. Steele et al., "Sexual Desire, Not Hypersexuality, Is Related to Neurophysiological Responses Elicited by Sexual Images," *Socioaffective Neuroscience & Psychology* 3, no. 1 (January 2013): 20770, https://doi.org/10.3402/snp.v3i0.20770.

94. Dawn M. Szymanski et al., "Sexual Minority Women's Relationship Quality: Examining the Roles of Multiple Oppressions and Silencing the Self," *Psychology of Sexual Orientation and Gender Diversity* 3, no. 1 (March 2016): 1–10, https://doi.org/10.1037/sgd0000145.

95. Samuel L. Perry and Cyrus Schleifer, "Till Porn Do Us Part? A Longitudinal Examination of Pornography Use and Divorce," *Journal of Sex Research* 55, no. 3 (May 2017): 284–296, https://doi.org/10.1080/00224499.2017.1317709.

Violent behavior is another topic that comes up when people discuss the dangers of porn. Does hardcore porn cause viewers to become more violent? A systematic[96] review of fifty-nine studies from the last twenty years found an association between excessive porn use and nonsexual violence, intimate partner sexual assault, and coercion. However, I want to note that correlation does not imply causation, so we don't actually know if hardcore porn causes people to be violent—but the association can mean that people who are violent tend to watch a lot of porn. What can we do to prevent this? Well, mindfulness is the key to every behavior and interaction. A mindful person isn't violent. If you feel like you're becoming reliant on violent porn, I'd recommend trying sexual meditation and guided masturbation audio porn to switch gears and find sexual stimulation in relaxation.

One of the most insidious dangers of porn is setting unrealistic expectations. I've seen this happen so much among both singles and couples. Some people learn about sex exclusively from mainstream porn, so their understanding of what to do during sex (e.g., aggressive constant thrusting, hair-pulling without asking, not wearing a condom), what sex should look and sound like (e.g., the female must look sexy and helpless while the male dominates, the female sounds feminine and young, the male doesn't make a sound), what the other person wants, and how desires and arousal work are colored entirely by scripted porn. Viewers who consume excessive amounts of porn may subconsciously internalize what sexual interactions "should" look like and therefore develop unhealthy or unrealistic expectations of sex in real life. This is why it's so important to educate people about porn literacy.

Early exposure to porn can be a form of sexual trauma, and it's important to seek professional help if you feel it's negatively affecting your intimate life. I stumbled on internet porn when I was about thirteen years old, but I was lucky enough to never encounter the really hardcore stuff,

96. Gemma Mestre-Bach et al., "Pornography Use and Violence: A Systematic Review of the Last 20 Years," *Trauma, Violence & Abuse* 25, no. 2 (June 2023): 1088–1112, https://doi.org/10.1177/15248380231173619.

like gang bangs or rape fantasies. I was watching videos of women getting fingered, which eventually became one of my favorite sexual activities. However, I can't say the same for all the other kids who stumble on porn when they're young and impressionable. I know that for many people, the porn they saw at a young age traumatized them. Researchers have identified that adolescents' porn viewing is potentially associated with more sexual aggression[97] and psychological distress.[98]

Finally, one of the most damaging types of porn is revenge porn. This occurs when a bitter previous lover publishes homemade sex photos or videos on the internet without the approval or knowledge of their ex-partner. It's illegal yet scarily prevalent. This is why I always tell people they need to be really careful who they make their kinky home videos with—you never know where they may end up. If your videos end up on the internet, make sure you report the other person to the authorities!

AFTERCARE OF PORN CONSUMPTION

When you watch porn, you're immersed in a different world—usually one that is full of fantasies and extra stimulation. This is why it's good to check in with yourself and your partner afterward. Self-care and partner-care after consuming porn is a necessary part of mindful and healthy behaviors.

For self-care, check in with yourself by responding to these questions:

- **How are you feeling after watching porn?**
- **Did anything specific trigger you to watch it?**
- **Are you experiencing any guilt or shame?**

---

97. Jochen Peter and Patti M. Valkenburg, "Adolescents and Pornography: A Review of 20 Years of Research," *Journal of Sex Research* 53, no. 4–5 (March 2016): 509–531, https://doi.org/10.1080/00224499.2016.1143441.

98. Caroline Giroux, "Early Exposure to Pornography: A Form of Sexual Trauma," *Journal of Psychiatry Reform* 10, no. 15 (December 2021): https://journalofpsychiatryreform.com/2021/12/07/early-exposure-to-pornography-a-form-of-sexual-trauma/.

- **Were the contents you watched mild, moderate, or intense?**
- **Were you able to be mindful and present during masturbation?**

For partner-care, check in with each other by asking and responding to these questions:

- **How are you feeling after watching porn?**
- **Did anything specific trigger you to watch it?**
- **Is there anything you need from me right now?**
- **Do you feel comfortable discussing your feelings about it?**
- **How can I best support you in this process?**

Remember, not all porn is your enemy, and you can actually use the different types, categories, and genres of porn to your advantage. I personally love exploring new things by watching ethical and instructional porn. In any given week, you'll find me spicing it up with my husband by watching some creampies and amateur videos, turning myself on by listening to audio porn and ASMR, and honing my sexual imagination by reading erotica. All these activities contribute to my very well-rounded and fulfilling sex life. So what are you watching, reading, or listening to tonight?

Chapter 11

How Outdated Norms Fucked Us All and How to Unfuck Ourselves

Sexuality should be celebrated, not hidden or shamed.

—Dr. Ruth Westheimer

Mary is an Asian American woman in her thirties with a fun, outspoken, tomboyish personality who has been struggling with dating for a long time. When she showed up to our first coaching session, she got right to the point: "I just want to start by saying I'm not here to get sex coaching. I'm here because you seem to have found a way to be a boss lady while being sexy and feminine. I see you're married to the love of your life, and I heard you guys talking about your relationship on your podcast. That's what I want: a life partner. I just can't seem to find or keep one, and I want you to analyze me. What's wrong with me?"

My first impression was "Wow, this woman is cool! She doesn't fuck around, and she gets right to the point!" I was a bit taken aback at first, though, because people usually come to session not really knowing exactly what they want to work on, but I loved Mary's energy and decisiveness. I never had a client like that before—someone who just shows up and declares, "I want what you have. Can you show me how to get there?"

I responded to her empathetically, "I don't think anything is wrong with you, Mary, but like I tell all my clients, we all have room for improvement, and only the brave ones want to tap into it. You're brave because you're here. I understand you like a no-BS, straightforward style of coaching, so I'll give that to you. No handholding. How does that sound?"

She immediately said, "That's perfect."

Over the course of three sessions, I learned that Mary had a lot of limiting beliefs regarding what a "good woman" should and shouldn't be. She was an assertive woman, but when she went on a date, she pretended to be someone else completely because of what her mother taught her: that she needs to act more "feminine" and "reserved" when she talks to men because she will be perceived as more attractive to them.

"You're too masculine," her mother used to tell her. "No boys will like you." In our sessions, we worked to unpack her true self and her sexual profile. Even though she said she wasn't there for sex coaching, I told her that she couldn't separate herself entirely from her sexuality. That's not how nature works. Your sexuality is within you, and you can either work against it or work with it to your advantage. For me, my sexual confidence fuels my life, career, relationships, and bank account.

Once we were able to establish a more consistent understanding of self, Mary was excited to learn that she had "natural feminine qualities." As we talked about other aspects of her life, I pointed out that she was very caring and nurturing with all her friends. That was far more representative of natural feminine qualities than being quiet in front of a man. Over three months, we worked on helping her feeling comfortable with herself and allowing her true personality to shine as her sexual confidence grew. Mary understood that her mom's beliefs, which she inherited, were outdated and soon overcame the toxic idea that she was too masculine for a good man. She learned to embrace her tough side while expressing more of her natural femininity. She learned to allow her dates to set up dinner (in the past, she would just volunteer to do it), let them take the lead in planning (in the past, she'd just tell them when and where to meet), and let them pick her up if they offer.

One time in the past, she asked a date, "Why are you coming all the way here to get me? It's out of your way and so inefficient." I pointed out that she belittled their good intention to provide convenience and comfort.

"If you can, accept it and thank them for their chivalry," I told her. "If you don't want to accept it, thank them and tell them you'd prefer meeting at the restaurant because it's easier." She nodded and looked like she had a lot to think about.

After a month or so, she came in with a smile and shared, "I went on a third date with this guy, Tommy, and I think it's going really well! He thinks my toughness is endearing. I told him about you and our sessions! He said he enjoys my quirks, and I feel the same about him. I think we're going on a little road trip to Santa Barbara this weekend. He planned the whole thing! I'm excited to get intimate. There's so much spark between us. Thank you again for everything."

She emailed me a few weeks after that to say that they were dating exclusively and that she wanted him to get some sessions with me because he has a hard time talking about his emotions. In our first session, I learned that he grew up in a loving family with a tough military dad who provided everything for him—except emotional safety. We're now working to undo the misguided idea that "real men don't talk about their feelings," which will be a bit of a journey.

Can we just admit it? So many outdated cultural and social norms regarding sex, dating, and relationships have really fucked us (and not in a good way). Gender norms from my grandmother's era (e.g., women should be subservient to their husbands, men shouldn't talk about their feelings) are outdated and fucking toxic. These "norms" have caused so much pain and problems in contemporary society. If you grew up as a boy, you might have heard things like "man up" or "real men don't cry," which is absurd because you're completely shutting out a perfectly healthy way to deal with emotions. Crying isn't inherently bad or a gender-based activity. It's actually not bad at all. Most of the time, it's a good release for everyone. If you grew up as a girl, you might have heard things like "be sweet and nice" or "don't be too assertive" because society likes a sweet girl who's feminine and accommodating. This is also ridiculous since it gives girls such limiting beliefs about what they can accomplish. You can totally be nice and kind while also being assertive and outspoken. It's not like you can only choose to be one thing. We are all multidimensional, and the more we accept that fact, the more we're able to live authentically and fully.

There's so much evidence[99] that shows certain outdated ideas don't work and cause unhappiness, a lack of advancement, and even mental health issues. Not all traditional views are terrible, though. Some people believe in happy and sexually fulfilled monogamous marriages, and I've witnessed that truth in many couples (but I've also seen lots of problematic ones). In our society, there tends to be shame toward everyone, which is horrible and unproductive. Shame if you want to become a housewife or stay-at-home dad. Shame if you don't want to have children. Shame if you fuck a lot of people. Shame if you don't have enough sex. Shame if you're stuck in a marriage where you're not fucking. Shame if you get a divorce. Shame if you talk about your feelings. Shame if you want an unconventional life. Shame if you want a traditional life. It seems like we can't win.

However, I truly believe we can, and if younger generations shift to be more understanding, accepting, and sex-positive, things will change and cultural norms will be adapted to what works for them. Less shame, more love (and orgasms), hopefully! So, can I be a bad bitch with a 401(k) and still be a sexual woman who gets taken care of in bed and at home by my loving and emotionally expressive husband? Fuck yeah, I can. This

99. Simon Rice et al., "Gender Norms and the Mental Health of Boys and Young Men," *Lancet Public Health* 6, no. 8 (August 2021): 541–542, https://doi.org/10.1016/s2468-2667(21)00138-9; Ruth Gaunt, "Breadwinners vs. Caregivers: Why Outdated Family Roles Are Bad for Everyone," in Essays on Equality: The Politics of Childcare, ed. Becca Shepard and George May (King's College London, 2023), 71–74.

chapter is about how some old-school norms have fucked us all, men and women, and how we can unfuck ourselves.

BULLSHIT WE DON'T NEED: FIFTEEN OUTDATED SOCIETAL AND CULTURAL NORMS

Sex before marriage is shameful.

It's terrible that this is still a thing. The belief that people can only have sex after getting married, that sex before marriage is shameful and you're probably going to hell if you're doing it, or that sex is only pure and right when it's between married heterosexual partners is honestly so harmful. Sex before marriage is normal. Sexual compatibility is a big part of overall relationship satisfaction, so how would you know it if you don't try? The shame narrative is so strong that a lot of religious young adults have to suppress their natural sexual desires and resort to "sex loopholes" like soaking (inserting the penis in the vagina without moving it in and out) and dry humping (nonpenetrative humping).

Purity[100] culture—abstinence or "staying pure" before marriage—is not a positive thing; it actually has adverse effects on young adults (e.g., mental health issues, stress and anxiety, panic attacks, low self-esteem, body image issues, inability to experience pleasure). Allowing young adults to safely explore their sexuality at their own pace without guilt and shame helps them grow a stronger sense of self-assurance and

[100] K. R. Griffin, "An Examination of the Association of Religiosity, Purity Culture, and Religious Trauma with Symptoms of Depression and Anxiety" (PhD diss., University of Nevada, Las Vegas, 2023); Katie Cross, "'I Have the Power in My Body to Make People Sin': The Trauma of Purity Culture and the Concept of 'Body Theodicy,'" in *Feminist Trauma Theologies: Body, Scripture and Church in Critical Perspective*, ed. K. O'Donnell and K. Cross (SCM Press, 2020), 21–39; Alyssa C. Jones and Jordyn M. Tipsword et al., "Fear of Sin and Fear of God: Scrupulosity Predicts Women's Daily Experiences of Mental Contamination Following Sexual Trauma," *Journal of Traumatic Stress* 36, no. 5 (August 2023): 932–942, https://doi.org/10.1002/jts.22961; Elizabeth Gish, "'Are You a "Trashable" Styrofoam Cup?': Harm and Damage Rhetoric in the Contemporary American Sexual Purity Movement," *Journal of Feminist Studies in Religion* 34, no. 2 (2018): 5, https://doi.org/10.2979/jfemistudreli.34.2.03.

sexual agency. If you grew up with purity culture at the forefront of your adolescent life, know that it's never too late to work on accepting and loving your sexuality. Working with a purity culture–informed coach and/or therapist, as well as reading and educating yourself more about human sexuality, can help you feel more capable and confident. If you have children, make sure you teach them that sex is normal and healthy, and provide a safe space for them to talk to you about it. Statistically, the typical age of sexual debut is sixteen to seventeen years old, so make sure you teach your teens to be safe and communicative. Using an empowering approach can help build a strong foundation for high self-esteem and good judgment when selecting a romantic and sexual partner. Fear-based communication about sex only drives your children away because they don't feel like you're a safe person to talk to about this kind of stuff—and that will cause way more problems in the future.

Good women are submissive. Real men are dominant.

If you don't already know, I'm not a submissive person. I know how to embrace my feminine qualities; how to be nurturing, kind, and empathetic; and how to ask for help when needed, but I'm not submissive or subservient. Some people are naturally more submissive, and that's OK! As long as it comes from an authentic and empowering place, there's no right or wrong way to be. I'm not here to shame anybody for their qualities.

The bullshit is that there's so many negative perceptions of women who are outspoken and assertive and of men who are reserved and passive. "She's such a bitch" is regularly used to describe women who exhibit themselves in a more dominant fashion than some people can stomach. Likewise, "He's such a pussy" is sometimes used to describe men who are not stereotypically dominant. Whether you're more masculine or feminine, everyone has positive qualities and flaws, and one isn't better than another. Masculinity and femininity exist in all of us.

Research[101] revealed that people who possess both traits tend to have better psychological well-being and health, so it's not a binary—it's more like a continuum. On a scale of 1 (not masculine at all) to 10 (extremely masculine), I'm probably a 5. I have many traits that would be considered masculine, like being assertive, straightforward, possessing leadership qualities, and protective, but not at an intense level. For femininity, on a scale of 1 (not feminine at all) to 10 (extremely feminine), I'm probably a solid 7. I'm emotionally expressive, caring, nurturing, empathetic, and collaborative. Where are you on the continuum?

Like Mary, many of us are still stuck with the outdated norm that "women should only be feminine and men should only be masculine." I hope this section helped you understand that whether you're more submissive or dominant, we all have feminine and masculine traits in us that should be celebrated and nurtured, and our levels of masculinity and femininity shouldn't overshadow simply being a good person and partner.

Real men don't talk about their feelings.

It doesn't matter what your gender is, talking about your feelings is very healthy. Suppressing[102] your emotions and not expressing them can cause mental, psychological, emotional, relational, and physical harm. Emotional intelligence is the ability to understand and manage your emotions positively. For example, being able to identify when you're angry, the cause of your anger, and managing your anger constructively so you don't explode on yourself and others is important. When you're emotionally intelligent, you're able to communicate your emotions more

101. M. Pilar Matud, "Masculine/Instrumental and Feminine/Expressive Traits and Health, Well-Being, and Psychological Distress in Spanish Men," *American Journal of Men's Health* 13, no. 1 (February 2019): https://doi.org/10.1177/1557988319832749.
102. Brett Q. Ford et al., "The Psychological Health Benefits of Accepting Negative Emotions and Thoughts: Laboratory, Diary, and Longitudinal Evidence," *Journal of Personality and Social Psychology* 115, no. 6 (July 2017): 1075–1092, https://doi.org/10.1037/pspp0000157.

effectively, empathize with others and their situations, experience less stress, and manage conflict in a productive way. Continuing to believe that "real men don't talk about their feelings" is toxic and problematic for both individuals and society. Research[103] found that men who have low emotional intelligence are more likely to be violent toward their wives and that low emotional intelligence is related to aggression.[104]

So what can we do? First, we need to teach everyone to embrace healthy emotional expressions. Suppressing it doesn't work. I encourage my husband to identify his emotions and talk about his feelings. I show him that I'm a safe space by withholding any kind of judgment toward how he's feeling and validating his emotional experiences. It's so important that we all learn to manage and communicate our emotions, both women and men, so we can feel empowered, heard, and supported. For people who do not get support from their partners when it comes to talking about their feelings, I highly recommend seeing a relationship coach or marriage counselor. Sometimes with a third-party intervention, people can gain new perspectives about their skills and limitations.

Long-term couples don't have sex.

So many couples have accepted this societal norm because it's so prevalent in the media. Consequently, it may be one of the main culprits for divorce and long-term relationship dissatisfaction. The human needs for sexual connection and wanting to feel desired don't just go away when we get older. Yes, it's common to experience lower libido as you age—especially for women older than fifty and men older than seventy—but I've seen couples in their thirties who have been married for only five

103. T. Jafarian, M. Fathi, M. Arshi, and R. Ghaderi, "The Effect of Men's Emotional Intelligence on Violence Against Women Among Married Couples," *Knowledge & Research in Applied Psychology* 16, no. 4 (2017): 76–83.

104. E. García-Sancho et al., "Relationship Between Emotional Intelligence and Aggression: A Systematic Review," *Aggression and Violent Behavior* 19, no. 5 (September 2014): 584–591, https://doi.org/10.1016/j.avb.2014.07.007.

years who no longer have sex. The lack of sexual connection is also one of the most common reasons why people engage in infidelity. The old saying "If I don't get it at home, I'll get it somewhere else" has some truth to it, but it's a toxic way of thinking about how to deal with sexual frustrations and relationship dissatisfaction.

If you feel sexually dissatisfied in your monogamous relationship, you should talk about it and work on a solution together. Yes, it will be hard at first, but if you don't talk about it, someone will inevitably cheat or just emotionally explode, which has such negative effects on both partners' mental and physical health. We don't have to accept the sexless marriage/relationship norm. Long-term couples' intimacy behaviors are associated with sexual satisfaction,[105] so yes, you can have a great sex life in a long-term relationship. We can be proactive in keeping our relationships fulfilled and connected, happy and joyful, exciting and communicative. All these things are possible when you put in the effort.

Only penetration counts as sex.

I believe this sexual norm is one of the main reasons why a lot of people in long-term relationships are sexually dissatisfied. When only one activity counts as "sex," it's extremely limiting and not at all fulfilling for long-term couples. Imagine being in a relationship with the same person for forty or fifty years and only vaginal penetration is considered "good sex." Nah, I don't think so.

Most people say, "Our sex life is boring," when I ask about the one sex issue they experience in a long-term relationship. Sexual exploration is key to a fulfilling long-term relationship. I'm not saying everyone should try going to a sex party or having a threesome—I use the term *sexual*

---

105. Noémie Beaulieu et al., "Toward an Integrative Model of Intimacy, Sexual Satisfaction, and Relationship Satisfaction: A Prospective Study in Long-Term Couples," *Journal of Sex Research* 60, no. 8 (October 2022): 1100–1112, https://doi.org/10.1080/00224499.2022.2129557.

exploration in a broad sense—but maybe you try a new sex toy together, a finger in the butt, sexual meditation for couples, or sexy board games. Don't get fixated on how to reclaim the spark you had when you started dating; that's being unrealistic. However, I advocate for sexual creativity and expanding your definition of good sex. When you have a variety of acceptable forms of "good sex," you allow yourself and your partner to become more sexually fulfilled by accepting pleasure in all its shapes and forms. Unfuck yourself by changing your perspective on what counts as sex.

Women are gold diggers and only want rich men.

Wanting financial stability in someone you date and being a gold digger are two totally different things. Any guy who argues otherwise is probably just insecure about their current financial situation and projecting. It's true that women tend to rate men with financial stability as more attractive and desirable than men without financial stability.[106] That just makes sense in the most basic human need way; people need resources to survive and thrive and for the health of their offspring, so of course women prefer to date men who are financially stable. They feel safe and secure with the freedom to explore unique experiences.

By contrast, a gold digger is in a relationship with someone for one sole purpose: to extract money from them. There's no love or care involved. This is completely different from women who are healthily dating and hoping to find love and a life partner. Nowadays, there are more women graduating from college than there are men[107], and although they're not getting paid at the same rate as men still, most women I

---

106. Devendra Singh, "Female Judgment of Male Attractiveness and Desirability for Relationships: Role of Waist-to-Hip Ratio and Financial Status," *Journal of Personality and Social Psychology* 69, no. 6 (1995): 1089–1101, https://doi.org/10.1037/0022-3514.69.6.1089.

107. Richard Fry, "Women Now Outnumber Men in the U.S. College-Educated Labor Force," Pew Research Center, September 26, 2022, https://www.pewresearch.org/short-reads/2022/09/26/women-now-outnumber-men-in-the-u-s-college-educated-labor-force/.

know are financially stable and thriving. It's reasonable that most of them want an equal partner.

However, some financially successful women don't have that kind of desire. Their priorities are different. I have one client who's a big baller attorney looking for a house husband. Even so, she finds it hard to find her true love. Many men she's dated were intimidated by her and probably preferred women who were not as financially secure. I hope we, as a society, can move past this BS norm and focus on establishing a new norm: "It's normal to desire a financially responsible partner."

Penis size is everything.

"Eight-inch big, ooh, that's good pipe"—Saweetie, "My Type"

"Extra large and extra hard"—Cardi B, "WAP"

"Can you get it up? Is you big enough?"—Rihanna, "Rude Boy"

There's so much messaging about penis size in pop culture. It's safe to say we're big-dick obsessed, to the point where I think it's giving a lot of guys really bad sexual anxiety and low self-esteem. I'm not saying size doesn't matter at all, because it does, but not as much as most men think. One study[108] surveyed more than fifty-two thousand straight men and women and found 85 percent of women were satisfied with their partner's penis, regardless of the size. However, only about half the men were happy with their dick size. About 45 percent wanted their penis to be bigger. Do you see the discrepancy?

The size issue doesn't just stay in the bedroom. Research[109] suggests men who think their penises are bigger than average tend to think they're

108. Janet Lever et al., "Does Size Matter? Men's and Women's Views on Penis Size Across the Lifespan," *Psychology of Men & Masculinity* 7, no. 3 (July 2006): 129–143, https://doi.org/10.1037/1524-9220.7.3.129.

109. Natalie Amos and Marita McCabe, "Positive Perceptions of Genital Appearance and Feeling Sexually Attractive: Is It a Matter of Sexual Esteem?," *Archives of Sexual Behavior* 45, no. 5 (July 2016): 1249–1258, https://pubmed.ncbi.nlm.nih.gov/26857376/.

more attractive, so a man's general sense of self-confidence is affected by his own perception of his dick. But manhood and masculinity shouldn't be reduced to just penis size. I know, easier said than done because I don't have a penis, but for real, a big dick doesn't always translate to a good lover, an interesting person, or a nice human. If your penis is smaller than average (the average is around 5 inches erect), develop a strong personality, sense of humor, sense of security, self-assurance, and confidence. Groom yourself well, be a generous and competent lover, and be a gentleman. These are all much more attractive traits than the size of your penis. Let's leave the big dick norm behind and embrace big positive energy.

Marriages are the only valid long-term relationships. And you should have a wedding!

You don't need to get married. You don't need to have a wedding. The reason why both made sense back in the day was due to property ownership and the legitimacy of offspring. In today's world, and with the resources we all possess, it's not at all necessary to get married (unless you get tax benefits, then you do you). Listen, I'm not talking shit about marriages. If you've always wanted to get married and it's your dream, I don't judge you. After all, I'm married too! I met the love of my life, and we wanted to have a fun wedding. We got married in the museum where Brent had a solo show at the time (he's an oil painter), and it was very special. But it's also OK if you don't care about it or don't want to get married. It doesn't make you less than or unfulfilled.

I think our society is still biased and judgmental toward unmarried long-term couples. It's kind of like, "What's wrong with them? Why are they not married?" It's such a big norm that you'll often hear people ask, "When are you guys going to get married?" It's also pretty crazy how much money people spend on their weddings to live out their fairytale dreams.

The average[110] wedding cost is $33,000—for one day of your life! But the range is so much more. Some people spend from $100,000 up to several million for their wedding day. At the end of the day, if that's what you truly desire, then go for it! But I think as a society we need to lay off the pressure on unmarried long-term couples. Don't ask when they're going to get married or assume that everyone needs to have a wedding. Their relationship is valid as is.

You're not living a fulfilling life if you don't have children.

Not having children doesn't affect your overall happiness and well-being.[111] Women have been led to believe that their lives are not fulfilled until they have children. I'm not against children. I'd actually like to have them someday, but I do think there's too much stigma surrounding couples who choose not to have children. Consider the following conversation, which I overheard while out to dinner.

"But you won't know what it's like to be a mother," one woman said.

Another woman immediately chimed in, "It's unlike anything you'll ever experience. You're gonna miss out on such a vital part of womanhood."

The woman who presumably told her friends that she decided not to have children said, "Yeah, but Mark and I are gonna travel the world and live our best lives together. We have enough nieces and nephews. We don't want children!"

---

110. Kiah Treece, "Average Wedding Cost: How Much Should You Budget for Your Big Day?" *Forbes Magazine*, April 3, 2024, www.forbes.com/advisor/personal-loans/average-cost-of-a-wedding/.

111. Hans-Peter Kohler et al., "Partner + Children = Happiness? The Effects of Partnerships and Fertility on Well-Being," *Population and Development Review* 31, no. 3 (October 2005): 407–445, https://doi.org/10.1111/j.1728-4457.2005.00078.x.

This conversation made me feel uncomfortable because the women were invalidating their friend's choice, and the way they spoke sounded like they believed their own experiences were better and womanlier. That's just bullshit. Let's leave this norm behind and do what we want to do. Want to have a kid or a bunch of kids? Do it. Don't want to have kids? All good. Let's not judge other people's choices. It's hard enough being a woman. We really need to support one another!

Men who like getting pegged are gay.

First of all, nothing's wrong with being gay. Second, your butthole doesn't have a sexual orientation. It's a neutral body part. It doesn't love someone of the same sex or different sex or certain genders. Everyone has a butthole, and everyone should be able to enjoy the pleasure that comes with it without hiding or feeling guilty. In fact, straight men who enjoy pegging also benefit from increased pleasure, psychosexual arousal, and deep connection with their partners.[112] There are also benefits[113] for relationships in which couples work pegging into their sexual repertoire, such as increased trust, shared intimacy, communication, and mutual pleasure. It's all good if you know you definitely don't want to try it, even though it can bring you so much pleasure and no one's forcing you, but calling it out as gay is homophobic, misguided, and false. Shaming heterosexual men who enjoy pegging is also toxic behavior. This norm needs to go. Welcome to a sex-positive world where people get to enjoy whatever the fuck they want as long as it's consensual and everyone is minding their own business.

---

112. D. J. Williams and Lynnette Coto, "'Best Sex He'd Ever Had!': A Qualitative Analysis of 'Most Amazing' Pegging Experiences," *Journal of Positive Sexuality* 9, no. 2 (December 2023): 15–18, https://doi.org/10.51681/1.923.
113. D. J. Williams et al., "'It's Absolutely Intense, and I Love It!' A Qualitative Investigation of 'Pegging' as Leisure," *Leisure Sciences* (June 2023): 1–15, https://doi.org/10.1080/01490400.2023.2226669.

You should only date and marry someone of your own race.
Did you know that interracial marriage has only been legal in the United States since 1967? Are you shocked?! So, what this means is that about sixty years ago, my marriage (and *many* others) would have been illegal. That's ridiculous, stupid, and racist because deep down, we all know that love transcends all and it's not about someone's racial background. According to Pew Research Center [114], one in six newlyweds married someone from a different race or ethnicity. Living in Los Angeles, I see interracial couples everywhere I go. Even though interracial marriage has been legalized for more than half a century, the remnants of that cultural norm still exists in many subcultures within the United States and around the world.

When my husband and I visit rural areas in the United States, we still get a lot of "looks" that honestly make me feel uncomfortable. Back in the '90s, only 27 percent[115] of people over fifty approved of interracial marriage, so it seems like a lot of these folks may have passed on their beliefs to younger family members. Some people face more backlash than others. Relationships with a white woman and Black man face more prejudice than those with a white man and Black woman.[116] All in all, these toxic norms need to go. Love is love, and only love should be a priority, not some silly old-school norm of "dating people your own race."

114. Travis Mitchell, "1. Trends and Patterns in Intermarriage," Pew Research Center, May 18, 2017, www.pewresearch.org/social-trends/2017/05/18/1-trends-and-patterns-in-intermarriage/.
115. Veera Korhonen, "U.S. Approval of Interracial Marriage by Age Group 2021," *Statista*, July 5, 2024, www.statista.com/statistics/1405681/us-approval-of-interracial-marriage-by-age-group/.
116. Amelia Stillwell and Brian S. Lowery, "Gendered Racial Boundary Maintenance: Social Penalties for White Women in Interracial Relationships," *Journal of Personality and Social Psychology* 121, no. 3 (September 2021): 548–572, https://doi.org/10.1037/pspi0000332.

Monogamy is the only valid type of relationship.

We're more than a quarter of the way through the twenty-first century, we need to stop shoving "the standard" down people's throats. Every type of relationship is valid when it's full of love and based on intention, honesty, and understanding. Whenever I talk to super traditional, narrow-minded monogamous couples, they make it known that they think any form of open relationship is either immoral, just a phase, inferior to them, weird, based on just sex, not love, just for young people, not a real relationship, or for people who have commitment issues. They also say, "Oh, they just don't love each other enough," "That's just cheating," "They haven't found the one," or "I would never be able to do that; I love my partner too much!" I've heard it all.

These judgment-based comments mainly help the speakers feel better about themselves while not trying to accept variety or any kind of difference in relationship orientations that don't conform with their own. In my opinion, love is the most powerful driving force of all, and it can come in any shape or form as long as it's honest and consensual. When people say non-monogamous couples just want to cheat on each other, they really don't know what nonmonogamy is. There's probably way more honesty and communication than with traditional monogamy because everything needs to be communicated openly and up front.

I respect everyone who lives authentically and unapologetically, even though their way of life may be nonnormative. I've met the nicest polyamorous people, open relationship partners, swinging couples, and people in other types of consensual non-monogamous relationships that may not even have a specific label to describe them yet. As a society, if we can accept and support one another's choices, we can cultivate more love and understanding, which will in turn contribute to a much healthier society. It's not about forcing people to subscribe to monogamy or non-monogamy; it's about acceptance.

Casual sex is immoral.

The word *immoral* is often defined as "conflicting with traditionally held moral principles." So here's my question: Who came up with these traditional principles in the first place? I want to be clear; I'm not here to promote casual sex, and this book is not propaganda for hookup culture. I'm simply pointing out that some of these old-school norms are full of shit, usually sexist, and put way more stress and pressure on people without good reason.

When people are sexually empowered, they can make decisions for themselves in an intentional manner. Whether they want to have sex with one person or enjoy having sex with multiple people, it's their prerogative. There's so much shame toward sexually active women, especially. If you're an adult and want to sexually experiment in a safe and consensual way, why the fuck not? The concept of body count is inherently misogynistic. Men can have a lot of sexual partners and are praised for it, while women get chastised for having abundant sexual experiences.

Casual sex is simply sexual activity with a person you're not in a committed relationship with. There's no subtext to it, it's not inherently bad or good; it is what it is. I've had really nice and orgasmic casual sex experiences and some terrible ones, but I don't regret any of them. They all contribute to my life experience and inform my personal sexual preferences. If you don't participate in casual sex, it doesn't make you're a better or worse person. You can still have amazing sex with your one and only long-term partner. Let's unfuck ourselves by not shaming people if they want to fuck one person or multiple people for the rest of their lives.

Lube is shameful, and your pussy should be wet all the time.

This norm is pure bullshit. It makes so many women feel insecure and develop low sexual self-esteem. Sometimes your pussy just won't be wet, even if you're mentally turned on and horny. It's called arousal non-concordance and usually isn't something to worry about—so long as it happens from time to time. Maybe you have a bad lover who doesn't spend enough time warming you up, proceeds to stick his dick in, and then has the audacity to ask, "Why are you not wet?" It might not be their intention to rush the process; maybe they just didn't know any better (which is why sex education and honest communication are so important). Some men get really excited and want to stick it in too quickly. Even I have to occasionally remind my husband that I'm not ready yet and he needs to play with me more. There are also just terrible lovers who don't care at all, even after you communicate with them. If that's the case, you're better off without them. They don't respect you about this, and they will inevitably disrespect you in other aspects of life.

There are many factors that contribute to vaginal wetness. A healthy vagina is typically slightly moist. According to gynecologist Dr. Jen Gunter,[117] a healthy female produces 1 to 4 milliliters of vaginal fluids in a day. When women are aroused, the Bartholin glands produce more fluid—but not always. Arousal non-concordance happens when your mind and body are disconnected. As a result, your body doesn't respond to you feeling mentally horny or you may experience wetness even though you're not mentally horny. People who experience a lot of stress, have a hormonal imbalance, have mental or physical disabilities, have a history of trauma, or experience sexual anxiety may experience more common arousal non-concordance. Remedies include sex education, communication, trying new things, working on emotional intimacy, and using lube! Lube feels amazing. I truly believe everyone should own and use it.

Make sure you get regular checkups with your gynecologist for your vaginal health. If there are no physical issues related to your arousal non-concordance, it's likely a mental block, communication issue, or

117. Dr. Jen Gunter, "How Much Vaginal Discharge Is Normal? I Made a Roux to Demonstrate," Dr. Jen Gunter, May 6, 2017, https://drjengunter.com/2017/05/06/how-much-vaginal-discharge-is-normal-i-made-a-roux-to-demonstrate/.

relationship issue. Let's unfuck ourselves and stop thinking women need to be wet all the time. Here's your new belief: Lube is great for my sexual well-being!

Don't talk about sex on the first date.

I wholeheartedly believe this is an old-school norm that needs to be thrown away. We're acting like sex is wrong, sinful, taboo, and unacceptable when we say, "Don't talk about sex on the first date." Why not? Why is it inappropriate? Who decided that? How about we try something new, something we know contributes to long-term sexual and relational satisfaction? I believe there's a way to have a healthy conversation about sexual preferences, views, and perspectives on the first date.

OK, I'll compromise. If you're adamant about not discussing sex on the first date, you should definitely talk about it before you actually have sex with someone. We need to shift the perspective. Talking about sex isn't inappropriate, and it doesn't have to sound creepy. It's healthy and essential when done right. Questions like "What are your thoughts on sexual compatibility in the dating process?" "In your opinion, is sex important in a long-term relationship?" and "Would you describe yourself as kinky or more vanilla?" should be completely normal to ask during a first (or second) date.

HOW ARE YOU FEELING?

I know this is a lot to take in, but we need to understand how these norms have fucked us and how we can move forward to be more sex-positive, empathetic, and loving. I created the following list as a check-in point and a reminder for you. Remember, we can always take it slow. If you subscribe to any of those outdated norms, it takes time to gradually change the way you view sex, dating, and relationships. It's never too late, though!

Unfuck Yourself: The Checklist

- **You understand that sex before marriage can be a good thing because it helps you determine sexual compatibility, but you should still be cool with people who want to wait because it's their body, their choice.**
- **Good men and women are everywhere, and we don't need to use levels of femininity and masculinity to judge them.**
- **Healthy men are emotionally intelligent and talk about their feelings.**
- **Long-term couples have sex and need some form of sexual intimacy.**
- **All types of sexual activities count as sex.**
- **It's perfectly normal and reasonable for heterosexual women to desire men with financial stability.**
- **Men don't have to pay for everything.**
- **A big penis doesn't equal a high-value man.**
- **A marriage and a wedding are not required for a happy long-term relationship.**
- **Having children is great, but not having children is also great.**
- **Pegging is a pleasurable activity anyone can enjoy.**
- **People can date outside or within their own race; it doesn't and shouldn't matter.**
- **Monogamy is just one type of relationship, and all types of relationships are valid when they're loving and consensual.**
- **Casual sex is fine, and not having casual sex is fine too.**
- **Lube is fucking great.**
- **Talking about sex early in a relationship is not bad or taboo. It's a reasonable expectation, considering that sexual compatibility is a big part of a relationship's success.**

Chapter 12

Sexless Relationship? No, Thanks!: How to Cultivate Long-Term Sexual Desire

Never settle for mediocre sex. Keep exploring and experimenting.

—Sue Johanson

"I haven't had sex with my husband in five years," Linda shared in our first session. "He stopped initiating, and I just didn't know what to do. I've never felt so alone." This was like lightning through my heart because I know how hard it is to be in a relationship where you feel lonely and don't feel romantically or sexually desired or appreciated, regardless of your gender or sexual orientation. Unfortunately, sexual dissatisfaction in long-term relationships is a common phenomenon. Millions of people around the world are in sexless relationships and marriages, leaving them high and dry.

How common are sexless relationships, you ask? Well, statistics reveal that 15 percent[118] of marriages in the United States are sexless.

118. Jean H. Kim et al., "Sociodemographic Correlates of Sexlessness Among American Adults and Associations with Self-Reported Happiness Levels: Evidence from the U.S. General Social Survey," *Archives of Sexual Behavior* 46, no. 8 (March 2017): 2403–2415, https://doi.org/10.1007/s10508-017-0968-7.

Considering there are about 62 million married couples in the country, that's almost 10 million married couples who are not having sex (at least with each other; we don't know what people do outside their marriages). That's more than the population of Singapore! And that's just married people in the United States. The number is much higher if we factor in unmarried couples in long-term relationships and look at couples beyond the United States.

People often ask me, "Is it always bad to have a sexless relationship? Asking for a friend." Personally, for me, that's not the type of relationship I want to have, but technically, doesn't have to be bad. It's your choice, and it depends on how you feel about it. Some couples are completely happy and content not having sex because they truly don't care about sexual intimacy. They find pleasure in other types of intimacy. There are also asexual people who don't necessarily enjoy sex all that much. In these cases, it's not a problem at all. But most couples in sexless relationships find it distressing and want to be more sexually satisfied, feel more sexually desired, and improve their sex lives.

"We haven't had sex for a couple months because we've been busy. Are we in a sexless relationship?" That's a valid question! What's a sexless relationship anyway? The answer is subjective because for some people, only having sex once a month qualifies, whereas others may feel like six months or a year of not having sex would be considered a sexless relationship. Social scientists have defined it in many ways, but in a very general sense, it includes romantic couples who haven't had sex in more than six months by choice—meaning they just don't have the desire to have sex with each other or feel like they're too busy to have sex. Whatever the underlying cause or true reason, they just choose not to have sex.

The point here isn't to compare yourself with others or statistics. It all depends on how you and your partner feel. When it comes to sexual frequency and fulfillment, there really isn't a one-size-fits-all solution. Do you feel good, happy, and fulfilled in your relationship even when you don't have sex? If so, there's absolutely nothing wrong with your relationship. Sexual frequency doesn't negatively affect you; maybe you care more about other types of intimacy rather than sexual intimacy. On the other hand, do you feel undesired, unfulfilled, and not very happy in your relationship because of the lack of sexual connection and intimacy? If so, then yes, let's do something about it. Remember, quality over quantity is definitely the better play here. Having shitty sex multiple times a week sounds like a nightmare I never want to experience. Having great, pleasurable sex once a week sounds a lot more enticing for long-term success and happiness. And the quantity will be right when the quality is there.

Sexual problems are among the most prominent contributors to divorce and breakups. The hard truth is that people who are in sexless marriages think about divorce much more often than people who are having sex. I should know. I got married young to the most perfect guy on paper, and we had a lot of fun together, but it wasn't a passionate relationship. To be frank, I wasn't happy. I felt this void inside me because the passionless marriage was affecting every other part of my life. Getting a divorce from someone with whom I was not sexually compatible was one of the hardest things I've ever done emotionally. But it's never just about sex. It's always much deeper and more complex. People want to feel alive, desired, and activated in their relationships. When there's a lack of passion, it's like living life in black and white.

The good news is there are many scientifically proven ways to initiate, cultivate, and maintain a passionate sex life and sexual desires in a long-term relationship. We just have to care more and take meaningful action. That's what my current husband and I promised each other. Can you promise me you'll try? In this chapter, I'll share four things you need to do to cultivate long-term sexual desire (based on extensive studies) and ten exercises I call erotic solutions that you can do in your relationship to get you there.

FOUR ESSENTIALS FOR AN ORGASMIC SEX LIFE

Sexual Well-Being

It all starts with *you*. We need to hold ourselves accountable for our own sexual well-being. If we don't start learning more about our bodies, sexual preferences and boundaries, different sensations, and how we feel about our sexual self, we could have sex with the best lover in the world and it'd still be shitty or, at best, just OK. I had mediocre sex for a long time and didn't understand why I had low sexual desire. I just didn't really crave sexual intimacy. When I learned more about my sexuality, I realized, "Oh wait, it's not because I had a naturally low sex drive or too much stress but because I didn't put an effort into understanding my sexual self." From then on, my motto became *No Mediocre Sex*. I make sure to put in the effort—and that my partner does too.

Caring for your sexual health includes taking care of your physical, mental, emotional, and social well-being in relation to sexuality. Let's dive into each of these a bit further.

Physical: The basic requirement here is that there's no pain when you masturbate or have sex. The more holistic and pleasure-centered aim is that your body responds to touch in a pleasurable way, you're able to have various types of orgasms, and you know your erogenous zones well. You know which parts to touch and how to touch them to turn you on. This is a lifelong journey since your preferences can change over time. You might feel like you know your body really well, but it can change as you age, so it's important to revisit this part regularly. For example, when I was younger, I used to enjoy kissing with a lot of tongue. Now I don't. Little things like that can make a big difference in your sex life. That's why it's important for sexual conversation to be a regular feature of every relationship.

Mental and emotional: Does sex feel bad for you? Does it cause stress and anxiety? Is it emotionally draining? If your answer to any of these questions is *yes*, then you should investigate why. You can do this by taking time to be introspective and engage in self-reflection or by meeting with a sex therapist or sex coach. The bottom line is that sex should feel good mentally and emotionally. It allows you to feel connected to yourself and your partner. It should not cause short- or long-term mental or emotional harm.

Social: Is sex a point of tension in your relationship? Does it help you feel closer together or drive you apart? Sex—good sex, at least—helps you feel closer to your partner. If it drives you apart, it's time to reevaluate that aspect of your relationship and have a proper conversation. And remember to relax! Sorry if this sounds preachy, but we all need to be reminded every once a while (me included). It's hard to even have space to think about having sex when you're chronically stressed out. Find your favorite ways to relax and make space for them in your routine. For me, that means putting exercise and bath time on my calendar. A relaxed you is more likely to transform into an aroused and orgasmic you.

Excitement Outside The Bedroom

Articles about sex positions to try to make your sex life more exciting are helpful when you want to test out something different, but many people don't have the desire or motivation to try anything at all because their relationship is, frankly, boring. Before you get to the point of "exciting things to try in the bedroom," you need to include more excitement *outside* the bedroom. Think of your relationship as a fruit. Is it a juicy strawberry, a tangy tangerine, or a stale apple? If it's a juicy strawberry, orgasmic! Keep doing what you're doing! If it's a tangy tangerine with a hard exterior, can we peel off that layer to get to the juicy part? If it's a stale apple, then we need to find a way to grow a sweet and crispy apple tree, not just cover it in caramel. Remember, a healthy tree needs sunlight and *moist* and well-drained soil.

How do you get more sunlight (excitement) in your relationship? Vacations can be exciting, but not everyone can afford them, so here are some other fun things to up the excitement factor outside the bedroom. Try something you've never done, such as go on a new hike, visit a new farmers market, catch a show at a nearby theater, visit gardens, try a new sport, cook a new recipe together, watch or do improv, or have a cocktail/mocktail making competition at home. I also invite you to reminisce and revisit something you've done before that you loved. Consider how you can create these sunlight moments regularly, especially in terms of keeping your apple tree healthy.

Think of the moist soil as your sexual energy and the well-drained soil as good communication. How can we keep it moist outside the bedroom? Playful attitudes and actions. Shift your perspective and behaviors. We can have fun and be playful, make six figures, and be respected in our fields. These factors are not mutually exclusive. You don't need to be serious all the time to gain respect from people, especially your lover.

Here's something I do to get into a more playful mood and attitude after a stressful day at work: sexual meditation. A quick five-minute meditation uplifts my mood and helps me reset from work identity to lover identity. I highly recommend you do it before you get home. Another small fun thing you can do is write a playful note about why you find your partner attractive and leave it around the house (or send them a text). You don't have to be Shakespeare or Cardi B; just be you. Here's one of my favorites: "You have beautiful balls. I love your balls." It gets him giggling and keeps the sexual energy going. Find something that works for you and allows you to create a playful mood for yourselves.

What about ways to keep the soil well drained? It's important not to keep negative emotions and resentment bottled up. Learn to communicate and collaborate to come up with solutions together. Questions like "How do you like to relax and get in the mood? Is there something I can do to help?" and "What are some fun new things you'd like to try?

It doesn't need to be about sex. Just anything in life. Let's talk about it and see how we can make it happen." Remember, if you find it hard to start the conversation, there's no shame in the couples therapy game! Sex and relationship coaches and therapists can help you navigate hard conversations.

Space

Michaela Boehm, one of the wisest sex experts out there (and Will Smith's intimacy coach), taught me that the best way to cultivate long-term sexual desire for your partner is to keep space. Space can mean and be executed in different ways depending on your preferences and situations. For example, I have a client who has her own apartment in Manhattan and a house in New Jersey that she and her husband live in. She stays at the apartment when she wants to be alone and write her movie scripts or when she has an event or night out in the city. They love it, even though it's a controversial arrangement. Many of their friends think it's bonkers for married couples to have separate places, but the couple thinks it's great for maintaining their long-term passion. It gives them "days off" to miss each other.

That sounds awesome, but it's just not possible for many of us. So, what can you do to create space? First, think about micro spaces, which can be nail salon time with your sister, a night out with your friends, or yoga class by yourself. Many couples also have physical micro spaces at home where they can spend time apart. For example, my father-in-law loves working on cars in the garage, and my mother runs on the treadmill at home in her gym corner. It's a form of self-care for both of them. Micro spaces are helpful in creating a healthy space between you and your partner. Remember that it's important to clearly communicate how much time each of you need in order to be on the same page and not leave either of you feeling neglected or unloved. For instance, I might text my husband, "Hey love, I'll be going to the spa with my friend for two hours. I won't have my phone, but I'll message you when I'm on my way home." In some instances, he'll respond with his alone time request, "OK, babe! I think I'm gonna go paint for a few hours, but I'll be back in time to take you to dinner."

To open up this conversation more generally, you can say, "I've read that it's great for people in romantic relationships to have alone time. How do you feel about that? I'd love for us to have an open conversation and figure out what that might look like for us. I love spending time with you, and I think a little space can make our time together even sweeter." Ultimately, you don't need to see each other 24/7. It's true that you need time apart to miss each other, and it's worth the effort to be more intentional and carve time out for space. Remember, a passionate relationship is a long-distance marathon, not a sprint.

Erotic Solutions

Erotic solutions are sexuality-related activities that are meant to satisfy different aspects of your sexual desires. Statistics show that most people want to have a fulfilling sex life, but two-thirds of us don't know what to do or how to start. I'm a pragmatic sexpert, and I want you to have all the tools necessary for long-term passionate relationships, so review the following activities and do one, three, or all of them! Remember to stay open-minded. Some people show so much resistance to trying something new for their sexuality and sex lives due to social conditioning, what they were taught growing up, or past trauma, so they don't approach these with an open mind. That's when these erotic solutions don't really work.

These erotic solutions are exercises inclusive for all couples. Whether you're in a monogamous, monogamish, open, or polyamorous relationship, you can do these exercises, and whatever your sexual profile is, you'll find these erotic solutions naughty and refreshing! They take effort to do, but if you're both in the mindset of wanting to experiment, then you're already in the right headspace to gain full benefits from them.

So, here are ten erotic solutions you can try with your partner. Close your eyes, let go, and enjoy!

DON'T LET ME GO: INTENTIONAL CUDDLING

"When she touches me like she means it, her grip feels like she desperately wants me." "When he holds me and looks at me like I'm the most precious gem to ever exist, all is right in the world and I'm bursting with joy and warmth from the inside." *This* is the quality I want from intentional romantic touch. Touch is infinitely powerful. That's why there's a phenomenon called touch starvation or touch deprivation[119] where you don't get touched at all (or not as much as you used to), which can be detrimental to your physical, mental, and emotional well-being.[120] Touch-starved people may not sleep well or they may have a weakened immune system,[121] which fucks with your physical health. Another obvious effect is on emotional and mental health.

I want to clearly note that you can also feel touch starved in general due to lack of affectionate touch from loved ones, friends, and family. However, being touch starved in a romantic relationship means you're not feeling loved or desired by your partner. All these things contribute

---

119. Mayuresh Vasudevan Konda, "Social Touch: Investigating the Effect of Mediated Social Touch on Social Presence" (master's thesis, University of Twente, 2022), 1–72, https://essay.utwente.nl/92190/1/Konda_MA_EEMCS.pdf.

120. Michael Banissy, *Touch Matters: Handshakes, Hugs, and the New Science on How Touch Can Enhance Your Well-Being* (Chronicle Prism, 2023); Juulia T. Suvilehto et al., "Topography of Social Touching Depends on Emotional Bonds Between Humans," *Proceedings of the National Academy of Sciences* 112, no. 45 (October 2015): 13811–13816, https://doi.org/10.1073/pnas.1519231112.

121. Shilo Rea, "Hugs Help Protect against Stress and Infection, Say Carnegie Mellon Researchers," Carnegie Mellon University, December 17, 2014, www.cmu.edu/news/stories/archives/2014/december/december17_hugsprotect.html.

to higher stress levels, anxiety, and chances of depression. We already live in an anxiety-inducing world. To add another factor to our coping mechanism is just cruel. I personally can't imagine what life would be like if my husband didn't touch me or cuddle with me for at least a few minutes every day. If that's what's happening in your relationship, I'm sending you loving energy, and I encourage you to try this erotic solution. If not, it's still an amazing activity to do regularly.

What are the benefits to intentional cuddling? There are so many, where do I start?! One, we're social animals and touch is a part of how we socialize, so cuddling serves as a reminder that we're connected to someone else. Two, touch is a necessity in a romantic relationship. As you know, physical touch is a type of intimacy, but sexual intimacy also involves touch, so this activity hits two birds with one stone. Intentional cuddling can feel sexual and sensual if you allow it. Three, you'll find that slowing down and being mindful with your lover is a treat because you get to relax and both give and receive affection. Nonverbal affectionate communication like cuddling contributes positively to your physical and emotional health, as well as strengthening the relationship. Four, cuddling releases oxytocin, dopamine, and serotonin, so it leaves you feeling *really* good.

Prep: Be naked or wear minimal clothing so you can be skin on skin. This is obviously more personal than being clothed. If you have kids, try to do this when they can't interrupt your session. If you prefer, you can shower together beforehand, but that's not necessary. Some people enjoy the pheromones from not showering (namely, me and my husband).

Time: 15+ minutes. If you can do it longer, that's great, but fifteen minutes of intentional cuddling allows for connection and oxytocin release. (The positive effects of hugging occur within thirty seconds—affectionate touch is powerful![122]) This is controversial but if you're some-

122. Karen M. Grewen et al., "Warm Partner Contact Is Related to Lower Cardiovascular Reactivity," *Behavioral Medicine* 29, no. 3 (January 2003): 123–130, https://doi.org/10.1080/08964280309596065.

one who gets fidgety without knowing what time it is, I recommend setting a timer for thirty minutes with an alarm that has a nice soft sound (not a loud beeping that ruins the mood).

Mindset, Mantra, and Potential Outcomes: Stay open-minded to any possible feelings that might come up. Be as patient and committed to the process as possible. The mantra for this is "I am ready to give and receive affection." As a result of this exercise, you may feel more loved and desired by your partner, and vice versa.

Dos and Don'ts:

Do: Play pleasant music that you enjoy, light a candle as a mood setter, talk about positive things (e.g., "What are our personal and professional goals this year?" "What are the great things about our relationship?" "What are some small wins we should celebrate?)"

Don't: Turn on the TV (intentional cuddling is all about focusing on your partner so don't include a visual distraction), talk about negative things, or nag.

NAMASTE MY LOVE: SEXUAL MEDITATION FOR COUPLES

"Breathe in . . . breathe out . . . relax your neck . . . relax your jaw . . . now I invite you to touch your nipples." That's a short excerpt from my guided sexual meditation on YouTube. Sexual meditation is an amazing way to connect with your partner sexually. When people think of meditation, they usually think of Buddhist monks, people who do it for mental health, or a yoga practice, but meditation can be very sexual if you'll allow me to guide you.

Sexual meditation is like a regular meditation practice, but it focuses on sexual thoughts, feelings, and sensations. It depends on what you're in the mood for that day. You can focus on sexual thoughts where you and your partner think about the last time you had passionate sex with each other or a fantasy of what you want to do with each other. You can also say sexual affirmations like "You are an amazing lover," "Your cock/pussy feels so good," or "I love having you inside me/being inside you."

You can focus on sexual feelings and sensations where you take deep synchronized breaths while touching each other's erogenous zones. For example, meditate while massaging each other's pubic areas.

The point is for you both to experience uninterrupted relaxation and sexual connection. Some of you might be thinking, "This sounds too woo-woo for me." Well, lots of academic social scientific studies[123] found that sexual meditation can be extremely beneficial for your sex life. The specific positive results outlined in these studies were increased sexual desire, arousal, lubrication, orgasm, and sexual satisfaction.

Prep: Get naked and sit or lay down comfortably, hold each other's hands, and have your device ready and near you so you can press play on the guided meditation.

Time: 5–10+ minutes (definitely longer if you're an advanced meditator)

Mindset, Mantra, and Potential Outcomes: You need a relaxed and nonjudgmental mindset. The mantra for this is "I am ready to sexually and spiritually connect with my partner." As a result of this exercise, you will feel more relaxed and sexually connected to your partner. You might even get that giddy feeling of trying something new.

Dos and Don'ts:

Do: Approach it with a playful attitude (if you're too serious about it, then it defeats the purpose).

Don't: Mock the process or belittle your partner for wanting to try a mindfulness-based activity.

---

123. Jonathan G. Kimmes et al., "A Treatment Model for Anxiety-Related Sexual Dysfunctions Using Mindfulness Meditation within a Sex-Positive Framework," *Sexual and Relationship Therapy* 30, no. 2 (February 2015): 286–296, https://doi.org/10.1080/14681994.2015.1013023; Simone L. McCreary and Kevin G. Alderson, "The Perceived Effects of Practicing Meditation on Women's Sexual and Relational Lives," *Sexual and Relationship Therapy* 28, no. 1–2 (February 2013): 105–119, https://doi.org/10.1080/14681994.2013.770830; David Goldmeier and Ali Mears, "Meditation: A Review of its Use in Western Medicine and, in Particular, its Role in the Management of Sexual Dysfunction," *Current Psychiatry Reviews* 6, no. 1 (February 2010): 11–14, https://doi.org/10.2174/157340010790596508.

AH, AHHH! MOANING EXERCISE

This erotic solution is all about sounds. Sounds are sexy. That's why we listen to music to feel more sexually confident and why some of us like to play sexy songs when we fuck and make love. Most of us also love hearing our partners moan, so there's definitely something magical, carnal, and attractive about sounds. Some people have energy stuck in their throats, so letting it go through this audible exercise should help your body relax and feel more in tune with your sexual being.

In this erotic solution, you're going to moan out loud with your partner. Go through these three levels, making small grunts (level 1), a moderate moan (level 2), and a full animalistic moan (level 3). Then go through all three again two more times. Debrief and talk about this exercise afterward. You can talk about how you felt doing the exercise. The first time I did it, I felt very silly and we ended up laughing quite a bit, but it was a fun moment. Remember, it doesn't have to be serious. These exercises are meant to be done with playfulness in mind.

Prep: Be naked or wear comfortable clothing, have a glass of warm water nearby (or a hot toddy, however you like to roll), play instrumental music (something instrumental that feels sexy to you; you can also check out Dr. Tara's sexy playlist on YouTube), and sit down and face each other. Let go of the idea that you have to sound a certain way. Any type of energetic release from your throat is a gem in this exercise. Have some fun!

Time: 5–10 minutes

Mindset, Mantra, and Potential Outcomes: You need a relaxed and nonjudgmental mindset. The mantra for this is "I am ready to let go, have fun, and connect with my partner." As a result of this exercise, you will feel more energized and sexually connected to your partner.

Dos and Don'ts:

Do: Really let go and release tension from your throat through uninhibited moaning, make eye contact with your partner, laugh if you want.

Don't: Make fun of your partner's voice or the way they moan because it could deter them from losing their inhibitions or trying something new ever again (there's a difference between laughing together and laughing at someone).

WATCH US GET OFF: MUTUAL MASTURBATION

I love watching my partner jerk off. It's so hot to see him getting hard, and when he cums, he lets out an animalistic grunt. For the longest time, people used to think that it was weird to masturbate in front of your partner. A lot of people live in shame and rather than talk about it, they hide and secretly masturbate. Why is it so wrong to masturbate when you're in a relationship? Well, it's not wrong at all, but some people fear that it may mean their partner is not attracted to them anymore. This is not a gendered thing. Both men and women masturbate.

I've seen a husband get pissed at his wife because she masturbates a couple times a week. He thinks the vibrator is his competition, not realizing that it's the only thing keeping her sexual. I've also seen a girlfriend get upset because her boyfriend secretly masturbates a few times a week. Instead of feeling shameful, guilty, and unwanted, we should all shift our perspectives and support each other's sexual well-being by embracing mutual masturbation. You can do it together in the same space or send a video of you masturbating and orgasming.

Prep: If you're doing this together in the same space, then get naked and comfortable in bed, play some music you like, and start masturbating. Grabbing each other's body parts can be hot too. (Sometimes I'll use a vibrator with one hand and stroke his cock with my other hand for a little bit and he'll grab and squeeze my breasts.)

Time: 10–15 minutes

Mindset, Mantra, and Potential Outcomes: You need an uninhibited mindset. Focus on mindfully masturbating and experiencing the pleasure in your body. The mantra for this is "We are here to celebrate self-pleasure." As a result of this exercise, you will feel more connected with your partner because masturbation doesn't have to be a shameful thing you do in secret.

Dos and Don'ts:

Do: Focus on yourself and your own pleasure, add kink by watching porn together if that's your choice, let loose and moan when you're building to an orgasm, tell your partner "I'm gonna cum" (this may arouse your partner even more).

Don't: Judge your partner and the way they masturbate, disturb them by saying something that's not related to the process (i.e., don't try to have a conversation; this exercise is to focus on self-pleasure and reducing shame).

ALL HAIL THE QUEEN: PUSSY WORSHIP 101

So many women grew up with sexual shame because mainstream culture told them that good girls don't open their legs. The sex negativity or ignorance that girls experience growing up all bundle up into this ball of shame that they experience as adults—either vividly and consciously or subconsciously. That narrative, that good girls are innocent and sexually passive and bad girls are sexually assertive, has fucked with women's relationships, sexuality, and sexual self-esteem. On top of all that crap, female pleasure isn't visible in the media, so many women grew up without thinking about their own pleasure.

This exercise is all about accepting, loving, and receiving love for your pussy. As a woman, your task is to remain relaxed, stay open-minded, and keep your legs open. Your partner will massage your pubic area and pussy, smell and say nice things to your pussy (e.g. "Your pussy is beautiful"), lick your pussy the way you find pleasurable, and finger your pussy until you cum. (The last step is optional, but it's definitely one of my favorite parts of the process.)

Prep: Light some candles and play your favorite music (or not, silence is also OK), get naked, lay down, and prop your butt on a pillow. The worshipper goes through the steps outlined above, and the receiver doesn't have to do anything except receive with an open mind.

Time: 10+ minutes

Mindset, Mantra, and Potential Outcomes: The receiver should be open to a pleasure mindset. The giver should be in a giving and nonjudgmental mindset. The mantra for this is "I am ready to receive attention and pleasure" and "I am a proud pleasure giver." As a result of this exercise, you will feel more like the queen you are: a queen who deserves all the attention and pleasure.

Dos and Don'ts:

Do: Try to stay present as a receiver and don't worry about how your pussy looks, smells, or tastes, give verbal feedback if you want your partner to lick your pussy or finger you in a certain way, take deep breaths throughout the exercise.

Don't: Give unproductive feedback like, "You're not good at eating pussy" (unhelpful and can cause the giver to feel resentful) or "It's OK, you don't have to do that" because you feel bad being a receiver (sis, let them worship you for this session).

SPIRITUAL FUCK: A YAB-YUM EXERCISE

Have you ever heard of yab-yumming? It's a practice rooted in Eastern philosophy and tantra. Traditionally, this is where the male sits down with his legs crossed and the female wraps her legs around him, but the roles can be filled by any gender and sexual orientation.

This is one of the most intimate poses you can do with your partner because you're making direct eye contact, breathing onto each other, and wrapping your arms around each other—and your genitals are literally connected. As an erotic solution, this is not a sex position, so you don't need to have penetrative sex (but if that desire comes after the exercise, feel free to do so!). Once you get into the seated—yab-yum—position, synchronize your breathing while maintaining deep eye contact with your partner. You can do the 4-4-4 breathing practice together: inhale for four seconds, hold for four seconds, and exhale for four seconds. Repeat this at least ten times—or whatever feels right for you.

Prep: Get naked and sit in the yab-yum position.

Time: 5–10+ minutes (definitely do it longer if you practice breathwork all the time and your legs will allow you to do so)

Mindset, Mantra, and Potential Outcomes: You need a relaxed and playful mindset. The mantra for this is "I am open to spiritually and sexually connecting with my partner." As a result of this exercise, you will feel more sexually and spiritually connected to your partner. You may also feel increased sexual desire, and sex can feel more in-synch because you can synchronize your breathing.

Dos and Don'ts:

Do: If you can't get naked for some reason, it's still great to do this exercise with your clothes on. Follow the breathwork pattern together (it doesn't have to be 4-4-4 if there's a different pattern you like), set a comfortable temperature in the room (since you can get pretty hot in this position).

Don't: Do the yab-yum position if your legs and knees are not capable (try sitting on a chair instead), play loud music because the point is to hear each other's breaths, talk during the exercise.

YOU KNOW ME SO WELL! A PLEASURE-MAPPING EXERCISE

Pleasure mapping is a fun exercise you can do with your partner that will not only feel good because you're being touched, massaged, licked, and grabbed in different places but also is educational because you and your partner will learn way more about which parts of your bodies are more or less arousing than others and what type of touch you like for those body parts. We all have erogenous zones—places on your body that feel extra stimulating—and we all have different preferences. For me, kissing and licking the side of my neck feels very arousing and can make me super horny, especially when coupled with kissing and massaging my pubic area. One of my clients, Adam, loves it when his partner massages his butt. It consistently gives him an erection. For Adam, kissing on the neck doesn't feel arousing at all.

What about you? What kind of touch turns you on? In this erotic solution, you're going to take turns and pleasure map your partner for thirty minutes. I know it seems like a long time, but trust me, it's not when you do the whole exercise. Take a look at the following list of erogenous zones. For each area, try three to six different types of touch (e.g., caressing, massaging, grabbing, kissing, licking, nibbling); if you have other erogenous zones that are not on this list, let your partner know. The person being mapped should tell their partner how good each part and each type of touch feels by saying *no*, *yes*, or *fuck yes!*

1. **Scalp**
2. **Ears**
3. **Neck**
4. **Lips**
5. **Hands and fingertips**
6. **Inner arms**
7. **Inner wrists**
8. **Nipples**
9. **Chest**
10. **Stomach**
11. **Lower back**
12. **Pubic area**
13. **Genital area**
14. **Inner thighs**
15. **Taint**
16. **Butt and butthole**
17. **Behind the knees**
18. **Feet and toes**

Prep: Get naked and lay comfortably on your bed. You can have light music playing but nothing too loud or chaotic; remember, you want to focus on the sensations in your body.

Time: 30 minutes per person

Mindset, Mantra, and Potential Outcomes: You need an open and curious mindset. The mantra for this is "I am curious about my and my partner's bodies." As a result of this exercise, you will feel more sexually confident because you know way more about your body, what type of touch turns you on, your partner's body, and how to touch them. This self-awareness and understanding about your partner will make you feel a lot more confident as a lover. Instead of fucking like a rock star, you'll be fucking like a competent lover! It's amazing!

Dos and Don'ts:

Do: Take your time, have fun, focus on the sensations in your body, see what truly feels good, and take deep breaths throughout the session.

Don't: Rush or use judgmental language if your partner doesn't enjoy something (e.g., "You're so weird" if your partner doesn't like nipple play).

YOUR KING HAS ARRIVED: PENIS WORSHIP 101

Millions of men experience penis insecurity, regardless of size, scent, aesthetic, or performance. Roughly one in three men experience sexual anxiety and erectile dysfunction at some point in their lifetime. One way to show affection and help reduce your partner's insecurity is to worship his penis, so yes, this erotic solution is all about the penis.

In this exercise, the penis owner doesn't have to do anything except receive pleasure with an open mind. How is this exercise different from a regular hand job or blow job? It's more intentional. It will feel a bit more ceremonial, as the attention is all on your partner with no reciprocity expected. It can make the male partner feel more loved, desired, and sexy because you want to do this for them. As a giver, you will massage his pubic area and start stroking the dick (you can use lube if he wants), smell and say nice things to his dick (e.g., "Your cock is amazing"), lick his cock up and down and around while making eye contact and letting out soft grunts, and suck that cock until he cums in your mouth (for extra naughty bonus points, you can swallow). Ejaculating is optional and there should be no pressure because he might not be able to get hard, stay erect, or orgasm.

Prep: Light some candles and play his favorite music (or not, some men prefer no music so he can hear her licking and sucking sounds), get naked or wear lingerie he likes, and have his favorite lube nearby.

Time: 10+ minutes

Mindset, Mantra, and Potential Outcomes: The receiver should be open to being worshipped. It might feel uncomfortable at first, especially if you've never received pleasure without reciprocating, but you'll soon realize it's a great feeling just to receive. The giver should be in a giving and nonjudgmental mindset. The empowering thought I usually have is that I feel sexy and powerful for giving my partner pleasure. The mantra for this is "I am ready to be worshiped" and "I am amazing at pleasuring my partner's cock." As a result of this exercise, the penis owner will feel sexy and sexually confident and satisfied. The worshipper will feel like a badass pleasure giver.

Dos and Don'ts:

Do: Focus on the cock, give compliments, ask for feedback, be patient.

Don't: Rush the process or act like you're obligated to do this, focus on the erection (some men can't get hard during this process), expect that he will ejaculate.

TELL ME WHAT GIVES YOU AN ICK: A SEXUAL TURN-OFF EXERCISE

It may seem counterintuitive to learn more about the things that turn your partner off. You might think it's better to know what turns them on, right? Well, yes, but both are important. Knowing what turns your partner off will help you understand their sexual desires better and not do the things they find unappealing. Use the following questions and have an open conversation with your partner. You can answer with as many examples as you'd like; I'm just including some of mine as examples. Remember, don't do this in bed. Have this conversation in a nonsexual setting (like at a coffee shop, over dinner, or on a hike). Finally, always explain why each of these things is a turn-off so you create a deeper understanding and not just a laundry list.

- **What are your sexual turn-offs in nonsexual settings? *(Mine is when people are rude to service workers; that makes my pussy dry because it shows they're not compassionate.)***
- **What are your sexual turn-offs during foreplay? *(Mine is not enough kissing because it feels like a lack of affection.)***
- **What are your sexual turn-offs during penetrative sex? *(Mine is putting it in without making sure I'm wet enough because it shows you don't care about my physical well-being—and it can cause a painful tear in my pussy.)***

- **What are your sexual turn-offs right after sex? *(Mine is grabbing the phone and playing with it because it shows you're addicted to your phone, which is not attractive to me.)***

Prep: Prime your partner that the conversation will be about sexual turn-offs so they think about it in advance.

Time: 30+ minutes (but it can take as long you'd like; I've seen people spend two hours doing this exercise)

Mindset, Mantra, and Potential Outcomes: You need to be in an empathetic and compassionate mindset. Focus on actively listening and understanding your partner as well as sharing your authentic self. The mantra for this is "I can confidently share my sexual preferences" and "I am an empathetic listener." As a result of this exercise, you will learn so much more about each other's turn-offs so you don't consistently do the things that are obviously unattractive to your partner. This should enhance the sexual attraction you have for each other. It's possible that you partner may share something you've done before or something you like to do. A good response that can mitigate the awkwardness is "Thanks for sharing your turn-offs with me. I noticed that choking is a turn-off for you, and I've done it with you before, so I apologize. I'm going to try to not do that anymore." A response for something that you like can be "Thank you for sharing your authentic feelings. I noticed you said you don't like choking, but I actually find it to be quite a turn-on. Is there something we can do as a compromise?"

Dos and Don'ts:

Do: Be honest because honesty will benefit both of you in the long run, put effort into really reflecting on your sexual turn-offs, talk about why they're such turn-offs for you.

Don't: Lie or hold back, say "I don't know," criticize your partner and scare them from sharing their thoughts again (e.g., "You're just so uptight," "Everything is a turn-off for you"), talk about your dislikes specific to your partner (e.g., "You turn me off when you wear cargo pants").

SEXUAL CONNECTION COMMITMENT CEREMONY

When people take their marriage vows, they often say they take each other for better and for worse and "until death do us part." However, for millions of divorcees, it really became "until *sex* do us part." Committing to each other's sexual well-being is an essential part of a passionate long-term relationship. Sexual connection doesn't just happen or stay the same over time. You have to put in the effort to keep your sexual connection alive and thriving.

This exercise is all about keeping yourself and each other accountable to living sexually connected lives. Use the following template and say your sexual connection commitment vows to each other. I recommend doing this exercise once a year.

> *I, [NAME], promise to put in the effort to stay sexually connected with you, [NAME]. I will not ignore you. I will pay attention to you, your needs, and your desires. I will not let you feel lonely in our relationship. I will make sure we maintain our intimacy. I will let you know when I feel like I want more sexual intimacy instead of assuming you don't desire me. I will not resent you for wanting to try something new sexually. Instead, I will communicate my boundaries. Finally, I will show you and communicate to you that I desire you. I commit to positively contributing to our sex lives.*

Prep: Let's celebrate our sexual bodies by getting naked for this ceremony. Have your vows ready, hold hands, make deep eye contact, and recite the vow!

Time: 10 minutes

Mindset, Mantra, and Potential Outcomes: For this ceremony, you need to keep a loving and playful mindset. The mantra for this is "I am ready to commit to my partner sexually." This ceremony will help you remind yourself and each other to prioritize your sexual and romantic connection, which in turn contributes to a more fulfilling sex life and romantic relationship.

Dos and Don'ts:

Do: Commit to the process and have fun, be authentic, embrace your romantic side.

Don't: Be too serious, mock the process, do this exercise when you're drunk, do this exercise if you're just deceiving your partner.

Which erotic solution will you try first? Schedule them and check them off one by one!

Erotic Solution	When?	Completed?
Don't Let Me Go: Intentional Cuddling		
Namaste My Love: Sexual Meditation for Couples		
Ah, Ahhh! Moaning Exercise		
Watch Us Get Off: Mutual Masturbation		
All Hail the Queen: Pussy Worship 101		
Spiritual Fuck: A Yab-Yum Exercise		
You Know Me So Well! A Pleasure Mapping Exercise		
Your King has Arrived: Penis Worship 101		
Tell Me What Gives You an Ick: A Sexual Turn-Off Exercise		
Sexual Connection Commitment Ceremony		

Remember, erotic solutions are here for you to help maintain the spark in your relationship. Long-term relationships are a marathon, not a sprint. Together, you must find different ways to inject novelty and excitement into your sex life and relationship to keep it fresh, connected, and passionate. Review the checklist together and chat about where you want to start. Have an erotic day!

Chapter 13

A Bit More Than Monogamy: The Future Is Monogamish

Monogam-ish isn't prescriptive; it's a term I coined to describe my relationship. We're mostly monogamous, much more monogamous than not. But there is some allowance and wiggle room around the edges that we both agreed to that makes us both happy.

—Dan Savage

Ben and Ashley were monogamous for the entirety of their ten-year relationship. Ashley wanted to talk about ways to spice up their relationship, so when she showed up for her Zoom session, she seemed nervous but in good spirits.

"I listened to your podcast and there was an episode where you talked about your marriage and the sexual explorations you guys do together," Ashley explained. "I think it's so different and fascinating. I don't know if that's something my partner and I can do, but I want to learn more about it and hear your opinion on how it might work for us."

I was impressed by how articulate she was, which showed me that she'd been thinking about this for a while. "Sure thing! Let's talk about it," I said. "I'm excited to see how I can help. My first question is . . . how come your partner isn't on this call with you?" I probed out of curiosity because when couples want to try something new together, they typically both show up on the call. When only one person wants to try something new but is unsure if their partner would be down for it, only one person shows up. I was right.

"Well, I wanted to talk about this with you first before I bring it up to my partner, Ben. We've been together for ten years. We live together and have two fur babies. I love him to death, but I think we need some excitement in the sex department," she revealed. We spent the session talking about the history of their relationship, their current sexual routine (in her own words, "It's just the same thing every time"), various types of play parties that I know of, and some ways they could spark more passion in their relationship without including another sexual partner. She had many questions, and after our consultation, she seemed more comforted and confident. We left with the understanding that there are many different ways to reignite the playful passion in her long-term relationship with Ben without incorporating sex parties.

A few days later, they both showed up to a coaching session. After the pleasantries, Ashley declared, "So, I've asked if he would want to try going to a sex party. He didn't say no, but he said, 'I'm not sure if that's for people like us' and didn't really explain why."

At this point, I completely understood their situation. Ashley was curious and wanted to see what it was like. She came to see me for affirmation and wanted to know how to navigate the scene safely physically, emotionally, and relationally. Ben, however, was not on board—yet. He was hesitant (and rightfully so) because he was filled with uncertainty of what it entailed and what the ramifications of going to a sex party would be on their long-term loving relationship. Many people I've talked to about nontraditional sexual adventures are like this at first. They're hesitant but not a *no*.

Ben immediately responded, "Well, I mean, we're not, like, swingers or poly, you know? We're vanilla and have been together since our 20s. I feel like we'd just be, like, fish out of water or something." His response confirmed my suspicion that he had a misconception of what play parties are like and the kind of people who attend them.

I quickly debunked the myth: "My husband and I are not swingers or polyamorous. We're monogamish, but you know, quite a few partygoers I know are actually monogamous." Then I proceeded to explain the many misconceptions about swingers and sex parties.

I understand most people want to know exactly what happens there and whether they have to participate. The simple answer is no, you never have to do anything you don't want to do. Sex parties (at least the ones I've experienced) are the most consensual places in the world when it comes to nightlife activities. Party organizers consistently talk about consent communication and protocols. You literally have a higher chance of getting unwanted sexual advances in regular clubs and bars than at sex parties. Many monogamous couples attend them to hang out, vibe, make friends, enjoy voyeurism, and fuck each other in a different setting. Some couples become monogamish by involving another person once in a while but are still very much committed to their own relationship. This is known as being socially monogamous.

After three months of coaching sessions, Ashley and Ben decided to try going to a party in their city. Months went by before I heard from them again. Admittedly, I was a bit concerned, but I finally heard from Ashley. She told me all about their experiences at the play parties. They've been to a few since we last talked, and she said the first time was a bit awkward but it was still different and exciting. The most recent time they went, she kissed a girl, which turned into a makeout session that got her really horny. They said goodnight to the lovely woman, then went to the bathroom where she gave Ben an impromptu blow job. They ended the night making love at home, and Ben made her cum multiple times.

Ashley said they still talk about their experiences in disbelief because it was not something "people from my hometown would do."

"Not that you know of." I giggled and corrected her. She then told me that they now consider themselves monogamish since they've both made out with another person. She said it feels freer and more exciting than traditional monogamy.

"Couples that play together, stay together, right?" she laughed. We ended the call with Ashley saying she knew that challenges would come up as a monogamish couple and that she would be back with Ben for another session soon.

I left her with these parting words: "Always overcommunicate. It's the best way to mitigate misunderstandings and assumptions in any relationship."

I want to declare that this chapter isn't propaganda. I'm not trying to convince anyone to become monogamish. It's not like I get paid every time a couple becomes monogamish; this isn't some kind of multilevel marketing scam. It's just me talking from personal experience and professional knowledge. I'll review definitions, talk about research findings, and share interesting facts. We'll go over the differences between monogamy and monogamish, different categories of nontraditional relationships, and end with a fun "your-ideal-relationship" exercise. Hold tight and enjoy the ride!

WHAT EXACTLY IS MONOGAMY?

Monogamy,[124] in a scientific sense, is defined as the practice of having only one sexual partner at a time. In nature, there aren't many social animals

124. "Monogamy Definition & Meaning," *Merriam-Webster*, www.merriam-webster.com/dictionary/monogamy.

that practice monogamy. The list includes puffins, penguins, beavers, and humans. Focusing on the latter, there are two types of monogamy as I see it: social monogamy and sexual monogamy. Social monogamy means two people are committed exclusively to live together, share resources, complete various tasks together, and are known societally as a pair. Sexual monogamy means two people are committed to having sex only with each other, which includes all types of sexual activities (not just penetrative sex). Yes, monogamy definitely means you don't flirt with other people because that could suggest sexual interest. Social and sexual monogamy together equals a monogamous marriage or exclusive long-term relationship in most contemporary societies.

Technically, being monogamous has nothing to do with love, but people have attached romanticism to it. It's a commitment you make to one person to love them, take care of them, and fuck only them forever (or until you get a divorce). Many people looking for this kind of love—their one true love, soulmate, partner in crime, twin flame, spouse, or life partner—to spend the rest of their lives with monogamously. I think monogamy can be beautiful, comforting, loving, and heartwarming. I adore certain parts of monogamy.

There are also plenty of benefits of a healthy monogamous relationship or marriage. It's important to highlight that the key word here is *healthy* because unhealthy monogamy doesn't convey these benefits. Examples[125] can include more resources (like time and effort) being contributed to one relationship, comfort of having a committed partner to share life's moments with, a lower chance of sexually transmitted infections due to having one partner, morality[126] or the feeling that the

---

125. Hope Klug, "Why Monogamy? A Review of Potential Ultimate Drivers," *Frontiers in Ecology and Evolution* 6 (March 2018): https://doi.org/10.3389/fevo.2018.00030.
126. Amy C. Moors and Amanda N. Gesselman et al., "Desire, Familiarity, and Engagement in Polyamory: Results from a National Sample of Single Adults in the United States," *Frontiers in Psychology* 12 (March 2021): https://doi.org/10.3389/fpsyg.2021.619640.

relationship is morally appropriate and supported by society, and more parental care for offspring with two parents.

Let's be real, though. Monogamy isn't sacred or superior to other types of relationships. The word *sacred* was often associated with monogamy because it was supported by many religious beliefs and practices. But the truth is lots of people are hypocrites and speak of loyalty but behave dishonestly. Infidelity is a huge problem among monogamous couples, so many people (too many) who preach that they want to have sex with one person forever don't end up doing that at all.

About 21 percent of Americans—that's one in five people—have cheated on their partners[127], and this only represents the people who admit to it in a survey. I'm sure there are plenty more people doing it who are too ashamed to admit it publicly. Lying, hiding, and cheating don't sound sacred to me. As terrible as I see it was now, I've cheated—so I get it. I didn't have the courage to have proper conversations with my previous partners, and the lack of honesty and integrity negatively affected my psychology and self-esteem. People's lives—and indiscretions—are much more complex than we know. From my personal experiences and professional observations, some people are not meant to be monogamous, but they try to do it to conform to what's socially acceptable.

It's time to accept this universal fact: Not everybody is meant to be in a monogamous relationship. And that's totally OK. Monogamy works well for some people, and that's great, but people should be able to design their own relationship as long as it's legal, consensual, and fulfilling for them.

MONOGAMISH?

"Humans have always been monogamous; it's the only way relationships work," said a man sitting next to me at a networking event as he

[127] Peter Moore, "1 in 5 Americans Say They've Been Unfaithful," YouGov, June 2, 2015, https://today.yougov.com/society/articles/12470-men-more-likely-think-cheating.

profusely claimed that his wife would never desire another man sexually. This argument is oh-so flawed. "People have always done this" or "It's always been this way" are examples of a basic logical misconception called tradition fallacy.

Humans used to chop people's heads off and put them on spikes around the city. It was always that way . . . until it wasn't. Women were not allowed to have a bank account in the past without their husband's approval. People always did that too; doesn't mean it was good. Obviously, not all traditions are great, and there are many we should definitely not continue to practice as the world moves forward.

When people say they want a "traditional marriage," do they really? Which part of the tradition do they want to partake in? What most modern couples fail to realize is that they're already in a nontraditional relationship if they both work and split the bills. Then there's the harsh reality that half the people who get married eventually get a divorce. Perhaps the old, "traditional" way of doing things doesn't really work for some people. That said, I've always loved certain parts of monogamy. My husband and I practice social monogamy wholeheartedly. I firmly believe he's my soulmate and that we'll spend the rest of our lives together. At the same time, we're also up for safe and fun sexual adventures that may include one or more other people if fitting opportunities arise. We know we can openly talk about it to prevent any misunderstandings, and it's so refreshing. We're not in an open marriage; we're monogamish. There's a difference.

I was a guest on a podcast one time, and the host asked me, "What the hell is monogamish?" He'd never heard the term before. "Isn't that like . . . cheating with some extra steps?"

"It's not cheating when both partners know what's going on," I explained. "It's honest and consensual. Cheating is when you're lying and hiding. This is the opposite of cheating; it's communicative and collaborative. We're monogamish so we're, like, 99 percent monogamous, 1 percent non-monogamous, which means we're open to sexual exploration with others from time to time."

Is that the same as being in an open relationship? Not exactly. It's a relatively new relationship term coined by sex columnist Dan Savage[128], but it's become quite popular because people feel like it explains their situation and what they desire more accurately than full-on monogamy or a completely open relationship. In short, it's monogamy most of the time but there's room for nontraditional naughtiness when the time is right and the context is appropriate. It's OK if you're skeptical. But I'm asking you to proceed with the rest of this chapter out of curiosity. Remember, you can always accept others and the way they live their lives without practicing it yourself. To each their own.

Based on my personal and professional observations, I believe the future is monogamish (or some form of flexible monogamy). We've been seeing a rise of open and polyamorous relationships in the last decade. One-third of Americans who participated in a 2024 study[129] reported having been in at least one non-monogamous relationship, and out of that group of people, about 21 percent were in a committed relationship that allows sexual exploration with others (i.e., monogamish).

Nevertheless, a majority of people still want to be in a relationship with one person and have one stable, loving partner. When I surveyed my Instagram followers, most people said they believe in soulmates, want to find their own version of "the one," and want to get married. I absolutely get it, and the beautiful thing about living in a sex-positive era is that we can kind of have both.

I'll be honest with you (as I've been in this whole book), I love erotic parties and sex clubs. I'm sexually adventurous but also wanted to get married, wear a poofy dress, and wake up next to the love of my life every single day forever and ever. Is that too much to ask? Not really. I'm in a

---

128. Dan Savage, "Monogamish," Savage Love, *Chicago Reader*, July 21, 2011, https://chicagoreader.com/columns-opinion/savage-love-monogamish/.

129. Carly Mallenbaum and Mimi Montgomery, "Polyamory Gets More Attention and Legal Protection," *Axios*, February 15, 2024, www.axios.com/2024/02/14/polyamory-laws-nonmonogamy-stigma.

monogamish marriage now with the man of my dreams. When I started living authentically and communicating my desires unapologetically, I was able to create the life I've always wanted by not denying my sexuality and still honoring the love and commitment I have for my partner—and you can too!

NONTRADITIONAL RELATIONSHIPS

First off, let me just say that I am not a nonmonogamy expert. I study these relationships, but it's not the focus of my entire academic career. I read the research and interview people who practice nonmonogamy on my podcast, but I wouldn't claim to be an expert on this topic. There are people who have written multiple books about it and have been in nonmonogamous relationships their whole lives, but that's not me. Think of me as your fun and informed friend who knows a few key things about nonmonogamy and wants to share.

Even though I have to explain a bunch of terms, I'm not a big fan of permanent labels. Things don't have to be permanent. You're allowed to change and grow as a result of your life experiences. I was a serial monogamist for a long time until I realized that I'm monogamish. I have a friend who used to be polyamorous but now is monogamous. So yes, terms help people organize their thoughts and understand how they and other people exist in the world, but they don't need to define you forever.

A traditional relationship (in a *real* traditional sense) is heteronormative and based on outdated gender roles and norms. For example, the husband is the breadwinner and provider, puts food on the table, is tough, initiates sex, and doesn't help out with chores because he's tired from working all day. Meanwhile, the wife is the household manager and caretaker, cooks and cleans, doesn't work outside the house (so she's financially dependent on the husband), and doesn't initiate sex. When it comes to sex, a traditional relationship is strictly monogamous in every way (but there was and still is plenty of cheating among "monogamous" couples).

Apart from monogamish, there are many types of relationships people practice that we can consider nontraditional. Maybe you split the bills. Maybe you're married but don't live together. Maybe you like going to sex parties together. Maybe you have a hall pass when you're traveling solo. Maybe you both work and split the household chores evenly. Maybe you love more than one person and are in a quad relationship. Maybe happy-ending massages are acceptable in your relationship.

The point of this chapter isn't to convince anyone to do anything they don't want to. It's to educate you about the relational diversity that exists in our society and normalize it. You don't need to subscribe to any of these categories; you can just create your own beautiful and fulfilling relationship. But categories can sometimes help people realize the type of relationship they want to be in, so let's get to learning more about them.

Egalitarian Relationships

In an egalitarian relationship, traditional gender roles are blurred. All the duties, obligations, and perks are shared by both partners. Both people contribute to the finances, household chores, life organization, sexual initiation, relationship maintenance, and decision-making processes. It may sound like most modern couples already do this, but that's not statistically true. According to Pew Research Center,[130] only 29 percent of marriages are considered egalitarian. Interestingly, research[131] has found that egalitarian partners reported having more sex with significantly

130. Richard Fry et al., "In a Growing Share of U.S. Marriages, Husbands and Wives Earn about the Same," Pew Research Center, April 13, 2023, www.pewresearch.org/social-trends/2023/04/13/in-a-growing-share-of-u-s-marriages-husbands-and-wives-earn-about-the-same/#:~:text=Marriages%20in%20which%20husbands%20and,from%20only%2011%25%20in%201972.

131. Daniel L. Carlson et al., "The Gendered Division of Housework and Couples' Sexual Relationships: A Reexamination," *Journal of Marriage and Family* 78, no. 4 (May 2016): 975–995, https://doi.org/10.1111/jomf.12313.

higher sexual frequency than conventional couples. Women in egalitarian relationships also had higher levels of relationship satisfaction compared to traditional relationships, but there's no significant difference for men.

Household chores can become one of the most vicious points of conflict in a long-term relationship and marriage, so I find it very interesting that a study[132] found that an egalitarian way of dividing chores can reduce and prevent spousal conflicts. Obviously, this doesn't mean that traditional relationships shouldn't exist or won't work and that everyone should become egalitarian (lots of people are happy with their traditional arrangement), but it's a call for an audit and evaluation of your current relationship to see if there are aspects of egalitarianism you can adopt to improve the passion and functioning of your present relationship.

I'd call my relationship semi-egalitarian because my husband makes more money than I do and provides financially for big things in life like our home, food, and travels, but I'm not fully dependent on him because I also work and have my own finances nicely set up. When it comes to decision making, we make most of them together through an honest and open discussion. We both have a voice, and no one dictates the relationship. As for chores, it's basically fifty-fifty. My husband loves to cook, and I try to help with the dishes. I vacuum, and he takes the trash out. We both do laundry. Honestly, I'm super happy with my setup. I can't imagine being married to someone who expects me to do all the chores because they are "wifey duties," but per usual, no negative judgment toward #tradwives. To each their own!

Househusband Relationships

People often joke about this type of relationship because it's unconventional and goes against so many gender expectations. Men are

132. Allison Daminger, "De-gendered Processes, Gendered Outcomes: How Egalitarian Couples Make Sense of Non-egalitarian Household Practices," *American Sociological Review* 85, no. 5 (September 2020): 806–829, https://doi.org/10.1177/0003122420950208.

traditionally seen as the breadwinners or primary income earners, but there's nothing wrong with this type of relationship at all if both partners are happy with the setup. According to Pew Research Center[133], the wife is the sole income earner in about 6 percent of marriages in the United States. While that number is low, it's still more than 18 million people, and the reality is they could be facing societal stigma daily for being in a nontraditional relationship. Research[134] indicated that the role of househusband is perceived more negatively than housewife. It's depressing that people can't cope with change, prefer for things to stay "the way it has been," and judge and criticize people who don't live in the past.

Househusband relationships can totally work with proper communication and honesty (like every other relationship). It's important to be aware of potential negative feelings that may come up and talk about them openly. Just like other types of relationships, there are always pros and cons.

Ethical Nonmonogamy (ENM)

You may have heard this term a few times in recent years. Ethical nonmonogamy (sometimes called consensual nonmonogamy) is an umbrella term for all types of non-monogamous relationships, and there are so many! Instead of explaining the specifics of their relationship, people might just say they're in ENM[135] for convenience purposes. ENM is defined[136]

---

133. Richard Fry et al., "In a Growing Share of U.S. Marriages, Husbands and Wives Earn about the Same."

134. Diane Keyser Wentworth and Robert M. Chell, "The Role of Househusband and Housewife as Perceived by a College Population," *Journal of Psychology* 135, no. 6 (November 2001): 639–650, https://doi.org/10.1080/00223980109603725.

135. Justin K. Mogilski et al., "Monogamy versus Consensual Non-monogamy: Alternative Approaches to Pursuing a Strategically Pluralistic Mating Strategy," *Archives of Sexual Behavior* 46, no. 2 (December 2015): 407–417, https://doi.org/10.1007/s10508-015-0658-2.

136. Olivia Guy-Evans, "Ethical Non-Monogamy: Basics & Rules for ENM Relationships," *Simply Psychology*, January 18, 2024, www.simplypsychology.org/what-is-ethical-non-monogamy.html.

as the practice of taking part in romantic or intimate relationships that are not completely exclusive. In ENM, partners talk about dating or engaging in sexual activities with others prior to it happening so it's consensual—and sometimes even appreciated. Appreciated, you say?! Yes, that's called *compersion*, which is the opposite of jealousy. It's what some ENM partners experience when they see their partners happy with someone else, whether it's via love or sexual gratification.

Research[137] found various benefits of ENM, including the ability to have your needs fulfilled by different partners, varied life experiences, sexual variety, increased excitement and satisfaction, personal growth/development, development of a loving community, and being more conscious of effectively communicating with your partner. A study[138] also found that partners in ENM relationships reported higher levels of sexual satisfaction and orgasm rates than monogamous couples.

But just like other types of relationships, it's not all sunshine and rainbows. Some documented[139] challenges of ENM involve lack of social acceptance, "coming out" to their families (many people say their families stop talking to them), time management, juggling family responsibilities, being an attentive partner, and teaching important values to children. I find the social stigma is hard to escape, especially for people who are socially non-monogamous (meaning they openly have more than one partner they see regularly). I sure hope the world is moving in a sex-positive direction and we let people do what they desire without being chastised as long as it's legal and consensual!

---

137. Amy C. Moors et al., "Unique and Shared Relationship Benefits of Consensually Non-monogamous and Monogamous Relationships," *European Psychologist* 22, no. 1 (January 2017): 55–71, https://doi.org/10.1027/1016-9040/a000278.
138. Terri D. Conley et al., "Sexual Satisfaction Among Individuals in Monogamous and Consensually Non-monogamous Relationships," *Journal of Social and Personal Relationships* 35, no. 4 (March 2018): 509–531, https://doi.org/10.1177/0265407517743078.
139. Milaine Alarie, "Family and Consensual Non-monogamy: Parents' Perceptions of Benefits and Challenges," *Journal of Marriage and Family* 86, no. 2 (December 2023): 494–512, https://doi.org/10.1111/jomf.12955.

Polyamory

About one in nine Americans[140] have been involved in a polyamorous relationship, a relational practice where someone can have multiple romantic partners (often within one group but not always). For example, three partners can date romantically or even be in a committed relationship with one another. This is called a *triad* or more commonly known as *throuple*. With four partners in the same setup, it's called a *quad*. There are many categories of polyamorous relationships. Let me explain some of the most common ones here.

Hierarchical poly means there's a primary partner you focus on and other secondary partners (metamours) you also love but don't spend as much time and resources with. The primary couple is the center of this relationship. *Nonhierarchical poly* means there isn't a primary couple in the group and everyone can negotiate their relationships however they want. *Parallel poly* means there is a primary couple and both partners can date outside their relationship but usually don't introduce their outside partners to each other. *Kitchen table poly* is the opposite arrangement; it's where all partners come together and discuss how to operate their relationships. *V poly* is when one person dates two people, but those two are not involved with each other.

Poly relationships can be open or closed. Fidelity in poly relationships usually follows the same rules as in monogamy. If you stray and engage in emotional or sexual infidelity with others outside the relationship, you're cheating. To have the capacity to love and take care of more than one romantic partner is an advantage not many of us have. Interestingly, research by the Kinsey Institute[141] found that there isn't a

140. Kinsey Institute, "Polyamory and Consensual Non-Monogamy in the US," Kinsey Institute Research Institute News, June 17, 2022, blogs.iu.edu/kinseyinstitute/2022/06/17/polyamory-and-consensual-non-monogamy-in-the-us/.

141. Amy C. Moors and Amanda N. Gesselman et al., "Desire, Familiarity, and Engagement in Polyamory: Results from a National Sample of Single Adults in the United States," *Frontiers in Psychology* 12 (March 2021): https://doi.org/10.3389/fpsyg.2021.619640.

"type" of person who's likely to be poly. Polyamorists can be Republican or Democrat, be low- or high-income earners, come from different racial backgrounds, and live anywhere in the country. If you feel like you might be poly, ask yourself, "Do I believe I can love more than one person at the same time? Am I OK with my partner having other partners as long as it's communicated prior? Would I enjoy having sexual relations with more than one partner?" If you answered *yes* to all three questions, you should investigate further by doing more research into polyamory (*Polysecure* by Jessica Fern and *More Than Two* by Franklin Veaux, Janet Hardy, and Tatiana Gill are great places to start).

Open Relationships

"I'm a comedian. I travel a lot for work. Sometimes I won't see her for months. Since we started dating, we knew that the best way to move forward being together was to be in an open relationship. It works amazingly. We've been together for many years now and I love her dearly."

What I've noticed is that an open relationship is really an effective arrangement for many couples in unique circumstances, such as people who travel a lot for work or have long-distance partners. Being in a monogamous long-distance relationship is challenging, so many couples opt to open up their relationships for a certain amount of time until they reunite. Like most relationships, partners in open relationships have rules that are discussed openly at the beginning of the relationship, but these rules can be adjusted as time goes by and both partners have more experience.

Research[142] found men are more inclined to open relationships. This makes sense when we look at it from an evolutionary psychology perspec-

---

142. Nichole Fairbrother et al., "Open Relationship Prevalence, Characteristics, and Correlates in a Nationally Representative Sample of Canadian Adults," *Journal of Sex Research* 56, no. 6 (April 2019): 695–704, https://doi.org/10.1080/00224499.2019.1580667.

tive. Men don't get pregnant, so the act of "sowing their seeds" has fewer life consequences than women who have multiple sexual partners. You may have heard people say, "Aren't all miserable couples trying to open up their relationships to spice it up?" Well, no. Levels of relationship satisfaction don't typically differ between open and monogamous couples. On the contrary, one study[143] indicated that partners in open relationships were happier than the general population. They also have more sex and are in better health. However, people in open relationships experience more societal stigma than people in polyamorous relationships. Again, one type of relationship isn't better than another. It all depends on you and your partner(s) and whatever feels the most authentic and fulfilling to everyone involved.

Swinging Relationships

"I don't think swingers truly love their partners," said a podcaster when I tried to explain that some people feel even closer to their partner after they start swinging. I wasn't taken aback when he said it because I've heard many such misconceptions and harsh claims about swingers before. Swingers get a lot of negative judgment from mainstream society, and research confirms this.[144] People often perceive swingers rather negatively, and many think swinging is irresponsible and immoral. So what's a swinging relationship? It's a committed relationship structure that allows for couples to engage in sexual activities with another couple(s). Formerly known as "wife-swap," the concept became well known in the 1950s and

143. James R. Fleckenstein and Derrell W. Cox, "The Association of an Open Relationship Orientation with Health and Happiness in a Sample of Older US Adults," *Sexual and Relationship Therapy* 30, no. 1 (November 2014): 94–116, https://doi.org/10.1080/14681994.2014.976997.

144. Jes L. Matsick et al., "Love and Sex: Polyamorous Relationships Are Perceived More Favorably than Swinging and Open Relationships," *Psychology & Sexuality* 5, no. 4 (September 2013): 339–348, https://doi.org/10.1080/19419899.2013.832934.

has consistently become more accepted—but it still experiences stigma and discrimination.

There are many benefits to swinging relationships.[145] Swingers report higher levels of sexual frequency and quality of sex, better variety to their sex lives, and stronger relationships. Do swingers have low self-esteem, leading them to seek validation from people outside their marriages? Nope. One study[146] looked at self-esteem among swingers compared to the general population and found that swingers have higher self-esteem! My belief is that the media has intentionally sensationalized the swinging lifestyle and that their day-to-day lives are not that different from most people's. Many swingers I've talked to find their lifestyle empowering, especially the women. Another misconception I hear often is that swinging is for "old people," but that's also not true. At swinging conventions, I've seen couples in their 20s and 30s, so people of various ages participate in this type of relationship.

All in all, whether it's swinging, being in an open relationship, loving multiple people in polyamory, practicing monogamish, or staying monogamous, all relationships are valid when it's consensual, happy, and fulfilling for everyone involved.

THE PROBLEM WITH OPENING UP YOUR RELATIONSHIP

"We've been fighting a lot, so we decided to open up our relationship," a client shared. That's a really difficult thing to hear as a relationship coach because I just know their relationship is likely going to end very soon (and it did, BTW). In this case, the underlying issue was the fact that they didn't work at maintaining romanticism and enthusiasm for each other.

---

145. Curtis Bergstrand and Jennifer Blevins Williams, "Today's Alternative Marriage Styles: The Case of Swingers," *Journal of Human Sexuality* 3 (October 2000).

146. Curtis Bergstrand and Jennifer Blevins Williams, "Today's Alternative Marriage Styles."

Therefore, by involving more people in their relationship, they didn't fix their problem but made it worse.

Becoming non-monogamous isn't something you do to fix a bad relationship. It will most likely make it worse and cause more misery for both partners. Sometimes it's better to just properly end the relationship. This is a problem I see a lot among people who are relationally and sexually uninformed.

"I think I'm poly," a friend said.

"What do you think it means to be poly?" I probed.

He hesitantly responded, "Um, I don't actually know, but I just don't think monogamy is for me."

After I shared a few relationship types that exist, we came to the conclusion that he actually wanted to be monogamish, not poly. Once he understood the differences, he proceeded to ask me if I thought his wife would be into that because she wasn't into the idea of poly. I told him I didn't know and that he shouldn't haphazardly tell his wife he wants something else like poly without knowing the actual definitions of the terms.

Non-monogamous relationships are as challenging as monogamous relationships; they both take work and require a lot of effort. You want to be in a non-monogamous relationship if it speaks true to you and feels authentic—when it feels fulfilling for you and is a loving, consciously chosen and communicative relationship, not when you're at the brink of divorce or breakup. Too many people have made that mistake, and their relationships still end in divorce. The annoying part is that they and society blame nonmonogamy for the relationship ending because that's the last thing they did to try to "save their marriage." Let's be honest, though: The relationship ended before they opened it up.

If you're curious about nonmonogamy, approach it with careful consideration, educate yourself on the subject, and go slow. Remember, you can always change your mind. We're not meant to experience everything we've ever wanted in our twenties.

DR. TARA'S YOUR-IDEAL-RELATIONSHIP EXERCISE

What follows are the primary aspects of a romantic relationship. Use this exercise to help you craft the kind of relationship that speaks true to you at this point in your life. Remember, people can change and grow based on their life experiences, so if you identified with one type of relationship in the past that doesn't feel authentic now, that's OK. You're allowed to change. Design your own relationship here and make sure you communicate openly with your partner(s). Always use empathy and compassion in these conversations.

Love and Emotional Commitment

Pick one of the following:

- **One and only person? (If the answer is *yes*, you can move on to the next topic.)**
- **Fully capable of loving two people?**
    - **How much emotional commitment for each person?**
- **Able to love many people?**
    - **How much emotional commitment for each person?**

Sexual Relations

Pick one of the following:

- **Only one person: my partner!**
- **Monogamish! What's OK? What's not OK?**
- **Fully open, free-range baby!**
- **Poly! Open or closed? Is sex OK with everyone in the relationship or just specific people?**

Financial Responsibilities

Answer all the questions:

- **Is there a sole or primary provider in the relationship? Who? How do they feel about it?**
- **Do you split finances 50/50, 70/30, 90/10? What do the finances look like in your relationship?**
- **Do you have a shared bank account? Individual bank account? Both?**
- **Who manages household finances like paying the bills?**

Family Planning

Answer all the questions:

- **Do you want kids? If *yes*, how many?**
- **Who's the primary caretaker, or is the work split evenly between partners?**
- **How do you want to raise your children?**
- **Who provides for the children financially?**

Household Management

Answer all the questions:

- **Who's responsible for which chores?**
- **Who books life appointments like doctors, dentists, and lawyers?**
- **Who plans and organizes travels, vacations, and trips?**
- **Who runs errands like going to the bank, going to the post office, and buying groceries?**

Time Commitment

Answer all the questions:

- **How much time is committed to your work?**
- **How much time is committed to your partner(s)?**
- **If you have children, how is time being allocated?**
- **How much time is committed to household chores, errands, and other responsibilities?**

Interests and Hobbies

Answer all the questions:

- **Do you have shared interests? Is it important that you have similar interests and hobbies? If *yes*, what are they?**
- **Do you each have individual interests? Is it important that you have different interests and hobbies? If *yes*, what are they?**

Social Networks

Answer all the questions:

- **Is it important to have a close relationship with your partner's family?**
- **Is it important that you and your partner(s) have mutual friends and spend time together?**
- **Is it important that your partner has no friends, a few friends, or a lot of friends?**
- **If heterosexual, is it OK for your partner to have friends of the opposite sex?**

Relational Communication

- **How often do you want to talk about the relationship? Pick one of the following:**
    - **Once a week**
    - **Once a month**
    - **Once every three months**
    - **Once a year**

After going through this exercise, you should have gained clarity on what you want in a romantic relationship and how you want it to function. Again, people grow and gain more life experiences that may or may not make us change our minds. This is why coming back to this list every year (or more often) is crucial so you can check and confirm if you still feel the same about everything. It's crucial to stay in alignment with your true passions and desires.

YOU'VE GOT THIS!

I hope you've found this chapter (and the entire book) interesting, inspiring, and empowering. I hope I've given you some empathy and support. I hope the information has brought clarity, curiosity, and expansion to your understanding of sexuality and romantic relationships. I'm a big fan of listening to and understanding various perspectives on sex, relationships, and romance, as well as accepting others for who they are—even if we don't agree. I think the world needs more social tolerance.

It's not you versus me; it's you and me and *all of us*. We can all have beautiful and thriving relationships in our own ways. Just imagine what would the world be like if everyone were in a healthy and sexually fulfilling relationship. Let's make it happen starting with *you*! Have an orgasmic day, my luv!

Conclusion

"Sexuality is one of the ways that we become enlightened, actually, because it leads us to self-knowledge."

—Alice Walker

Sex, in its purest form (or in an intentionally nasty way), is beautiful. It's not shameful, inappropriate, or taboo. It's an act of human connection, play, pleasure, and discovery. It can be a source of positive and powerful energy that expands and enhances every part of your life.

Sex sounds simple but constitutes a vast topic of study. I know that many topics in this book could be the subject of an entire book on their own. There's so much more to explore and discover. For instance, there are books about tantra, BDSM, polyamory, and so forth that dive very deep into each specific topic. If you're interested in learning more about any of the topics discussed in this book, I have a resource library for you to check out. *How Do You Like It?* is meant to be a survey of all these topics to help you better understand yourself—because self-knowledge is key to a successful relationship and a healthy sex life. To help you become the lover you want to be: one who feels authentic to you, one who communicates clearly, and one who is empowered by pleasure. If you ever feel disconnected with your sexuality or with your partner in the future, know that you can always come back to this book and find a point of inspiration or sexploration together.

Since I first embarked on my sexual empowerment journey, I've grown to be much happier, more content, and more self-assured. I even make more money, have better skin, got married to my soulmate and best friend, and have the most fulfilling relationship I've had in my entire life. However, when your sexuality is neglected, it can be the source of misery and discontent. But now you've read this whole book, so you already know that, you sexpert! You can harness your sexual energy in a positive or negative way—it's entirely up to you.

I wrote this book because I want to help you become more educated about sex and comfortable with your sexuality. I want to equip you with necessary knowledge so you can use it to make an informed decision for your own sex life. I've never been a fan of propaganda, and this book is not it. It's simply a nonjudgmental guide to having a great sex life according to your own definition. In this book, we traveled a long journey together, from understanding ourselves on deeper levels to learning the most important sex skills to sexual communication and discovering the impact of societal and cultural norms on our sexual attitudes, beliefs, and values.

Sex is not just about sex. Sex is about everything else. Recently, I had a fruitful conversation with a very wise friend on his podcast, and I came to realize that I've battled perfectionism and shame my whole life. Ultimately, I just want to feel *free*. Perfectionism makes you feel trapped. I got married to my first husband because I wanted to have a seemingly "perfect" life. We had a good friendship, but we didn't share sexual chemistry. When I decided to get a divorce, I was swallowed in shame—but at the same time, I had a glimpse of hope.

I recognized that it was time to design my life in a way that I truly desired. Throughout my life, I was hiding behind the shame of "I don't want to fit inside a box" because, as a woman, I was taught not to be "too much," "too loud," "too sexual," or "too assertive." I shouldn't be those things, but I am. I am all the things. I can effectively teach my students as a professor, speak at an academic conference, make social media content about eating pussy, and go to a sex party all in the same day. I can dress up in suits or skimpy little dresses, and both are powerful. I am multidimensional, and you are too!

I used to have a limiting belief that I needed to present myself a certain way to gain respect from others. But one day, I realized that when people say, "You don't look or sound like a professor," it's reflecting their limiting beliefs, not mine. Once I changed my views and actions to align with my authentic self, I felt free. I am free. I live my life to the fullest based on my own definition. To me, sexual empowerment is freedom. Speaking up for your own pleasure is freedom. Educating others about sex positivity so they can liberate themselves is freedom. Being in a sexually explorative relationship is freedom. It took me a while to get here, but my life is exactly how I want it to be. Fuck shame. Fuck being perfect. My sexuality is my power, and the more I embrace it, the more I feel limitless.

As I'm finishing up this book, I've done deep self-reflection and found myself relearning multiple lessons I've learned throughout many years of studying sex. There's *so much* in the world of sexuality for us to explore and try solo and with our partner(s). Who knows, maybe we'll be able to have a threesome with an AI robot sometime soon. It makes me feel hopeful that sex in a long-term relationship doesn't have to be boring. The power is in our own hands. The societal narrative of a sexless marriage doesn't have to be true. You can make your own truth if you get on the same page with your partner and put in the effort together. Make sexual connection one of your top priorities.

On this journey, you learned about:

- **Your sexual profile. I'm DKFA ("The Party Animal"), what about you?**
- **Your sexual self-esteem and sexual confidence. How do you feel about that now?**
- **Sexual mindfulness, why it's so important for a satisfying sex life, and how to become more sexually mindful with and without your eyes closed.**
- **Sex education for adults, since most of us have never had real sex ed.**
- **Your kinky side and common nontraditional sexual behaviors.**
- **Macro sexual communication and how to do it to improve your sex life.**

- **Micro verbal and nonverbal sexual communication. Now you can dirty talk!**
- **Sex technology and how to use it to your advantage.**
- **Your sexual fantasies, what they mean, and why you shouldn't be ashamed of them.**
- **Porn and understanding why it isn't the problem—sexual shame is.**
- **Outdated social and cultural norms that influence our negative beliefs about sex.**
- **Sexless relationships and how to avoid them.**
- **Different types of nontraditional relationships and why the future might be monogamish. It's just like monogamy, only a bit naughtier.**

Having a fulfilling sex life is a choice. You have to put in the effort to get it and maintain it. Learning more about your sexual self is a choice. Embracing your sexuality, desires, and preferences is a choice. Loving your body is a choice. Communicating about sex constructively with your partner(s) is a choice. Engaging in dirty talk, sexting, and sexual meditation is a choice. Spending time giving yourself pleasure is a choice. Becoming a competent lover is a choice. Honoring your sexual self is . . . I think you get it.

We make hundreds of decisions every day. When it comes to having a great sex life, you need to decide for yourself if you truly want it. Then you can decide what you will do to get it and maintain it because the road to sexual well-being is wonderful, long, and winding. You will encounter potholes, detours, speed bumps, and wild animals, but as long as you're in the driver's seat, you know how to stay on course and keep driving.

Acknowledgments

I'm so grateful for my amazing community, Luvbites, for all the brave individuals who share their stories and help uplift others to become more sexually enlightened and for everyone's continued support in my purpose—spreading sexual positivity far and wide—so we can empower everyone in the world. Massive thanks to my editor, Soyolmaa Lkhagvadorj, whose smile lights up all our book meetings and whose work on editing is perfection. Deep gratitude for my literary agent, Olga Filina, for believing in me and my vision from the get-go without questioning if it's "too much" or "too out there." My family, whose unwavering support for my well-being and success since I was born is the reason why I'm right here, right now, with the opportunity to create this book and help the world become happier and more fulfilled. Big thanks to my best friend, Megan Fisk, whose enthusiasm for this book has been the best reminder of why I needed to write it and share it with everyone. Thank you for your help and support, always. Of course, it takes a village to run our wonderful sex-positive community and write this amazing book, so huge thanks to my team members: Victoria, for organizing my whole life and never once questioning why we do what we do; Adam, for all my social media aspirations and of course for your astrological wisdom and always having great energy; and Abby, for being the best intern who took on the biggest task of formatting all the resources in this book. Finally, to my beloved husband, Brent Estabrook, THANK YOU for being you . . . my number one supporter, lover, partner-in-crime, best friend, soulmate, and forever love. You light my fire.

References

Chapter 1:

Kassel, Gabrielle. "20 Common Sexual Kinks, According to Sex Educators, and Why It's Totally Normal to Have a Kink." *Business Insider*, February 24, 2023. www.businessinsider.com/guides/health/sex-relationships/list-of-kinks.

Lehmiller, Justin J. *Tell Me What You Want: The Science of Sexual Desire and How It Can Help You Improve Your Sex Life*. Da Capo Lifelong Books, 2018.

Stanton, Glenn T. "What Is the Actual Divorce Rate?" *Focus on the Family*, November 4, 2015. www.focusonthefamily.com/marriage/what-is-the-actual-divorce-rate/.

Taylor, Jordyn, and Milan Polk. "1 in 3 US Men Are Kinkier Now than before Covid, Sex Survey Shows." *Men's Health*, February 14, 2022. www.menshealth.com/sex-women/a38912652/mens-health-kink-sex-survey/.

Chapter 2:

Barnum, Emily L., and Kristin M. Perrone-McGovern. "Attachment, Self-Esteem, and Subjective Well-Being Among Survivors of Childhood Sexual Trauma." *Journal of Mental Health Counseling* 39, no. 1 (January 2017): 39–55. https://doi.org/10.17744/mehc.39.1.04.

Flores, Dalmacio, and Julie Barroso. "21st Century Parent–Child Sex Communication in the United States: A Process Review." *Journal of Sex Research* 54, no. 4–5 (January 2017): 532–548. https://doi.org/10.1080/00224499.2016.1267693.

Ford, Fae Diana. "Exploring the Impact of Negative and Positive Self-Talk in Relation to Loneliness and Self-Esteem in Secondary School-Aged Adolescents." PhD diss., University of Bolton, 2015.

Gam, Rahul Taye, et al. "Body Shaming Among School-Going Adolescents: Prevalence and Predictors." *International Journal Of Community Medicine And Public Health* 7, no. 4 (March 2020): 1324. https://doi.org/10.18203/2394-6040.ijcmph20201075.

Jones, Jeffrey M. "LGBT Identification in U.S. Ticks up to 7.1%." *Gallup*, March 14, 2024. news.gallup.com/poll/389792/lgbt-identification-ticks-up.aspx.

McClintock, Karen A. *Sexual Shame: An Urgent Call to Healing*. Fortress Press, 2001.

Mellor, David, et al. "Body Image and Self-Esteem Across Age and Gender: A Short-Term Longitudinal Study." *Sex Roles* 63, no. 9–10 (July 2010): 672–681. https://doi.org/10.1007/s11199-010-9813-3.

Prabhu, S., and D. D'Cunha. "Comparison of Body Image Perception and the Actual BMI and Correlation with Self-Esteem and Mental Health: A Cross-Sectional

Study Among Adolescents." *International Journal of Health and Allied Sciences* 7, no. 3 (2018): 145–149. doi:10.4103/ijhas.IJHAS_65_16.
"Scope of the Problem: Statistics." RAINN. www.rainn.org/statistics/scope-problem.
"State of Sex Education in USA: Health Education in Schools." Planned Parenthood. www.plannedparenthood.org/learn/for-educators/whats-state-sex-education-us.
Tod, David, et al. "Effects of Self-Talk: A Systematic Review." *Journal of Sport and Exercise Psychology* 33, no. 5 (October 2011): 666–687. https://doi.org/10.1123/jsep.33.5.666.

Chapter 3:

Ayres, Joe, and Brian L. Heuett. "An Examination of the Long-Term Effect of Performance Visualization." *Communication Research Reports* 17, no. 3 (2000): 229–236. https://doi.org/10.1080/08824090009388770.
Brassard, Audrey, et al. "Attachment Insecurities and Women's Sexual Function and Satisfaction: The Mediating Roles of Sexual Self-Esteem, Sexual Anxiety, and Sexual Assertiveness." *Journal of Sex Research* 52, no. 1 (December 2013): 110–119. https://doi.org/10.1080/00224499.2013.838744.
Brotto, Lori A., and Rosemary Basson. "Group Mindfulness-Based Therapy Significantly Improves Sexual Desire in Women." *Behaviour Research and Therapy* 57 (June 2014): 43–54. https://doi.org/10.1016/j.brat.2014.04.001.
Brotto, Lori A., and Rosemary Basson, et al. "A Mindfulness-Based Group Psychoeducational Intervention Targeting Sexual Arousal Disorder in Women." *Journal of Sexual Medicine* 5, no. 7 (July 2008): 1646–1659. https://doi.org/10.1111/j.1743-6109.2008.00850.x.
Brotto, Lori A., and Yvonne Erskine, et al. "A Brief Mindfulness-Based Cognitive Behavioral Intervention Improves Sexual Functioning versus Wait-List Control in Women Treated for Gynecologic Cancer." *Gynecologic Oncology* 125, no. 2 (May 2012): 320–325. https://doi.org/10.1016/j.ygyno.2012.01.035.
Byers, E. Sandra. "Relationship Satisfaction and Sexual Satisfaction: A Longitudinal Study of Individuals in Long-Term Relationships." *Journal of Sex Research* 42, no. 2 (May 2005): 113–118. https://doi.org/10.1080/00224490509552264.
Dhikav, Vikas, et al. "Yoga in Female Sexual Functions." *Journal of Sexual Medicine* 7, no. 2 (February 2010): 964–970. https://doi.org/10.1111/j.1743-6109.2009.01580.x.
Dhikav, Vikas, et al. "Yoga in Male Sexual Functioning: A Noncomparative Pilot Study." *Journal of Sexual Medicine* 7, no. 10 (October 2010): 3460–3466. https://doi.org/10.1111/j.1743-6109.2010.01930.x.
"Dr. Lori Brotto: UBC Sexual Health Research: Mindfulness Expert." Department of Obstetrics and Gynaecology, University of British Columbia. brottolab.med.ubc.ca/.
Dunkley, Cara R., et al. "The Potential Role of Mindfulness in Protecting Against Sexual Insecurities." *Canadian Journal of Human Sexuality* 24, no. 2 (August 2015): 92–103. https://doi.org/10.3138/cjhs.242-a7.
Grace, Asia. "Your Partner Is Probably Fantasizing about Someone Else during Sex: New Study." *New York Post*, September 8, 2023. nypost.com/2023/09/08/almost-half-of-americans-think-about-someone-else-during-sex-study/.

"Harvard Second Generation Grant and Glueck Study." Harvard Study of Adult Development. www.adultdevelopmentstudy.org/grantandglueckstudy.

Hassan, Amir Khalid. "Relation Between Mouth Breather Patients and Their Sexual Activities, Pilot Study." *Journal of Oral Health and Dental Science* 3, no. 2 (May 2019): 1–3.

Jaderek, Izabela, and Michal Lew-Starowicz. "A Systematic Review on Mindfulness Meditation–Based Interventions for Sexual Dysfunctions." *Journal of Sexual Medicine* 16, no. 10 (October 2019): 1581–1596. https://doi.org/10.1016/j.jsxm.2019.07.019.

Jaderek, Izabela, Katarzyna Obarska, and Michal Lew-Starowicz. "Assessment of the Effect of Mindfulness Monotherapy on Sexual Dysfunction Symptoms and Sex-Related Quality of Life in Women." *Sexual Medicine* 11, no. 3 (June 2023): 1–17. https://doi.org/10.1093/sexmed/qfad022.

Leavitt, Chelom E., et al. "The Role of Sexual Mindfulness in Sexual Wellbeing, Relational Wellbeing, and Self-Esteem." *Journal of Sex & Marital Therapy* 45, no. 6 (March 2019): 497–509. https://doi.org/10.1080/0092623x.2019.1572680.

Prause, N. "Porn Is for Masturbation." *Archives of Sexual Behavior* 48, no. 8 (2019): 2271–2277. https://doi.org/10.1007/s10508-019-1397-6.

White, David Gordon. *Kiss of the Yogini: "Tantric Sex" in Its South Asian Contexts*. University of Chicago Press, 2006.

Chapter 4:

Furnham, Adrian, et al. "Waist to Hip Ratio and Facial Attractiveness: A Pilot Study." *Personality and Individual Differences* 30, no. 3 (February 2001): 491–502. https://doi.org/10.1016/s0191-8869(00)00040-4.

Herbenick, Debby, Tsung-Chieh Fu, Callie Patterson, and J. Dennis Fortenberry. "Exercise-Induced Orgasm and Its Association with Sleep Orgasms and Orgasms During Partnered Sex: Findings from a U.S. Probability Survey." *Archives of Sexual Behavior* 50, no. 6 (August 2021): 2631–2640. https://doi.org/10.1007/s10508-021-01996-9.

Chapter 5:

Eckstein, Monica, Gabriela Stößel, Martin Fungisai Gerchen, Edda Bilek, Peter Kirsch, and Beate Ditzen. "Neural Responses to Instructed Positive Couple Interaction: An fMRI Study of Compliment Sharing." *Social Cognitive and Affective Neuroscience* 18, no. 1 (February 2023). https://doi.org/10.1093/scan/nsad005.

Kallmann, Carolee A. "A Review of 'Insatiable Wives: Women Who Stray and the Men Who Love Them.'" *Journal of Sex & Marital Therapy* 36, no. 5 (September 2010): 449–451. https://doi.org/10.1080/0092623x.2010.512228.

Lehmiller, Justin J., David Ley, and Dan Savage. "The Psychology of Gay Men's Cuckolding Fantasies." *Archives of Sexual Behavior* 47, no. 4 (May 2018): 999–1013. https://pubmed.ncbi.nlm.nih.gov/29285655/.

Scorolli, C., et al. "Relative Prevalence of Different Fetishes." *International Journal of Impotence Research* 19, no. 4 (February 2007): 432–437. https://doi.org/10.1038/sj.ijir.3901547.

Ventriglio, Antonio, et al. "Sexuality in the 21st Century: Leather or Rubber? Fetishism Explained." *Medical Journal Armed Forces India* 75, no. 2 (April 2019): 121–124. https://doi.org/10.1016/j.mjafi.2018.09.009.

Chapter 6:

Byers, E. Sandra. "Relationship Satisfaction and Sexual Satisfaction: A Longitudinal Study of Individuals in Long-Term Relationships." *Journal of Sex Research* 42, no. 2 (May 2005): 113–118. https://doi.org/10.1080/00224490509552264.

Hatfield, Elaine, and Richard L. Rapson. *Love, Sex, and Intimacy: Their Psychology, Biology, and History*. HarperCollins College Publishers, 1996.

Jones, Adam C., et al. "The Role of Sexual Communication in Couples' Sexual Outcomes: A Dyadic Path Analysis." *Journal of Marital and Family Therapy* 44, no. 4 (October 2017): 606–623. https://doi.org/10.1111/jmft.12282.

Knobloch, Leanne K. "Uncertainty Reduction Theory." *The International Encyclopedia of Interpersonal Communication*, December 2015, 1–9. https://doi.org/10.1002/9781118540190.wbeic144.

MacNeil, Sheila, and E. Sandra Byers. "Dyadic Assessment of Sexual Self-Disclosure and Sexual Satisfaction in Heterosexual Dating Couples." *Journal of Social and Personal Relationships* 22, no. 2 (April 2005): 169–181. https://doi.org/10.1177/0265407505050942.

Mallory, Allen B. "Dimensions of Couples' Sexual Communication, Relationship Satisfaction, and Sexual Satisfaction: A Meta-Analysis." *Journal of Family Psychology* 36, no. 3 (April 2022): 358–371. https://doi.org/10.1037/fam0000946.

Montesi, Jennifer L., et al. "On the Relationship Among Social Anxiety, Intimacy, Sexual Communication, and Sexual Satisfaction in Young Couples." *Archives of Sexual Behavior* 42, no. 1 (April 2012): 81–91. https://doi.org/10.1007/s10508-012-9929-3.

Oattes, M. K., and A. Offman. "Global Self-Esteem and Sexual Self-Esteem as Predictors of Sexual Communication in Intimate Relationships." *Canadian Journal of Human Sexuality* 16, no. 3 (January 2007): 89–100.

Suwinyattichaiporn, Tara. "Become Sexually Powerful." TEDx CSUF, Fullerton, CA, December 2, 2021. 11 min., 9 sec. www.youtube.com/watch?v=u-tkbBnmfbw.

Chapter 7:

Babin, Elizabeth A. "An Examination of Predictors of Nonverbal and Verbal Communication of Pleasure During Sex and Sexual Satisfaction." *Journal of Social and Personal Relationships* 30, no. 3 (August 2012): 270–292. https://doi.org/10.1177/0265407512454523.

Bennett, Margaret. "Talk Dirty to Me: An Examination of the Effects of Communication During Sexual Activity on Relational Outcomes for Young Adults Beginning

Romantic Relationships." PhD diss., University of Connecticut, 2019. https://digitalcommons.lib.uconn.edu/dissertations/2209/.

Blunt-Vinti, Heather, et al. "Show or Tell? Does Verbal and/or Nonverbal Sexual Communication Matter for Sexual Satisfaction?" *Journal of Sex & Marital Therapy* 45, no. 3 (April 2019): 206–217. https://doi.org/10.1080/0092623x.2018.1501446.

Denes, Amanda. "Gene X Environment Interactions and Pillow Talk: Investigating the Associations Among the OXTR Gene, Orgasm, Post-Sex Communication, and Relationship Satisfaction in Young Adult Relationships." *Communication Studies* 72, no. 1 (August 2020): 68–65. https://doi.org/10.1080/10510974.2020.1807373.

Denes, Amanda. "Pillow Talk: Exploring Disclosures After Sexual Activity." *Western Journal of Communication* 76, no. 2 (March 2012): 91–108. https://doi.org/10.1080/10570314.2011.651253.

Lutmer, Audrey, and Alicia M. Walker. "Patterns of Verbal and Nonverbal Communication during Sex." *Archives of Sexual Behavior* 53, no. 4 (April 2024): 1449–1462. https://pubmed.ncbi.nlm.nih.gov/38361172/.

Chapter 8:

Andersen, Kjeld V., and Gunnar Bovim. "Impotence and Nerve Entrapment in Long Distance Amateur Cyclists." *Acta Neurologica Scandinavica* 95, no. 4 (April 1997): 233–240. https://doi.org/10.1111/j.1600-0404.1997.tb00104.x.

Chen, Angela. "From Ice Age Dildos to VR, an Academic Explains the History and Future of Sex Toys." *Verge*, February 14, 2018. www.theverge.com/2018/2/14/17009834/hallie-lieberman-buzz-sex-toys-history-technology.

Gaboriault, Melanie. "What I've Learned About the New Era of Communication from my Gen Z Kids." *Fast Company*, December 11, 2022. https://www.fastcompany.com/90819951/what-ive-learned-about-the-new-era-of-communication-from-my-gen-z-kids.

Gordon-Messer, Deborah, et al. "Sexting Among Young Adults." *Journal of Adolescent Health* 52, no. 3 (March 2013): 301–306. https://doi.org/10.1016/j.jadohealth.2012.05.013.

Guess, Marsha K., et al. "Genital Sensation and Sexual Function in Women Bicyclists and Runners: Are Your Feet Safer than Your Seat?" *Journal of Sexual Medicine* 3, no. 6 (November 2006): 1018–1027. https://doi.org/10.1111/j.1743-6109.2006.00317.x.

Hald, Gert Martin, et al. "Do Sex Toys Make Me Satisfied? The Use of Sex Toys in Denmark, Norway, Sweden, Finland, France, and the UK." *Journal of Sex Research* (January 2024): 1–15. https://doi.org/10.1080/00224499.2024.2304575.

Johns, Sarah E., and Nerys Bushnell. "What Drives Sex Toy Popularity? A Morphological Examination of Vaginally-Insertable Products Sold by the World's Largest Sexual Wellness Company." *Journal of Sex Research* 61, no. 2 (February 2023): 161–168. https://doi.org/10.1080/00224499.2023.2175193.

Lindau, Stacy Tessler, et al. "A Study of Sexuality and Health Among Older Adults in the United States." *New England Journal of Medicine* 357, no. 8 (August 2007): 762–774. https://doi.org/10.1056/nejmoa067423.

Neustaedter, Carman, and Saul Greenberg. "Intimacy in Long-Distance Relationships Over Video Chat." *Proceedings of the SIGCHI Conference on Human Factors in Computing Systems* (May 2012): 753–762. https://doi.org/10.1145/2207676.2207785.

Paul, Pamela. "He Sexts, She Sexts More, Report Says." *New York Times*, July 15, 2011. www.nytimes.com/2011/07/17/fashion/women-are-more-likely-to-sext-than-men-study-says-studied.html?_r=1&src=recg.

Rubattu, Valeria, et al. "'Cam Girls and Adult Performers Are Enjoying a Boom in Business': The Reportage on the Pandemic Impact on Virtual Sex Work." *Social Sciences* 12, no. 2 (January 2023): 62. https://doi.org/10.3390/socsci12020062.

Schlott, Rikki. "Parents Reveal Teen Sons Committed Suicide after Being 'Sextorted': 'This Is Terrorism.'" *New York Post*, August 30, 2023. nypost.com/2023/08/30/parents-reveal-teen-sons-committed-suicide-after-sextortion/.

"Sex Toys Market Size, Share, Analysis, Forecast, Trend 2030." *Spherical Insights*, April 2023. www.sphericalinsights.com/reports/sex-toys-market.

Slutever. "Meet Harmony the Sex Robot." VICE TV, March 14, 2018. Video, 4 min., 33 sec. www.youtube.com/watch?v=orBH_Qnw3eY.

Spangler, Todd. "OnlyFans Payments Surged to Record $6.6 Billion in 2023, Up 19%." *Variety*, September 6, 2024. https://variety.com/2024/digital/news/onlyfans-payments-2023-financials-revenue-creator-earnings-1236135425/.

Tin, Jia Jian, et al. "Potential Benefits of Sexting Among Long-Term Monogamous Romantic Partners." *Journal of Counseling Sexology & Sexual Wellness: Research, Practice, and Education* 3, no. 2 (January 2022): 30–38. https://doi.org/10.34296/03021053.

Chapter 9:

Bivona, Jenny M., et al. "Women's Rape Fantasies: An Empirical Evaluation of the Major Explanations." *Archives of Sexual Behavior* 41, no. 5 (April 2012): 1107–1119. https://doi.org/10.1007/s10508-012-9934-6.

Bivona, Jenny, and Joseph Critelli. "The Nature of Women's Rape Fantasies: An Analysis of Prevalence, Frequency, and Contents." *Journal of Sex Research* 46, no. 1 (February 2009): 33–45. https://doi.org/10.1080/00224490802624406.

Hicks, Thomas V., and Harold Leitenberg. "Sexual Fantasies About One's Partner versus Someone Else: Gender Differences in Incidence and Frequency." *Journal of Sex Research* 38, no. 1 (February 2001): 43–51. https://doi.org/10.1080/00224490109552069.

Joyal, Christian C., et al. "What Exactly Is an Unusual Sexual Fantasy?" *Journal of Sexual Medicine* 12, no. 2 (February 2015): 328–340. https://doi.org/10.1111/jsm.12734.

Kahr, Brett. *Who's Been Sleeping in Your Head: The Secret World of Sexual Fantasies*. Basic Books, 2009.

Morris, Hannah, et al. "Three's a Crowd or Bonus?: College Students' Threesome Experiences." *Journal of Positive Sexuality* 2, no. 3 (October 2016): 62–76. https://doi.org/10.51681/1.234.

Psychology Today Staff. "Fantasies." *Psychology Today*. www.psychologytoday.com/us/basics/fantasies.

Williams, Kevin M., et al. "Inferring Sexually Deviant Behavior from Corresponding Fantasies: The Role of Personality and Pornography Consumption." *Criminal Justice and Behavior* 36, no. 2 (December 2008): 198–222. https://doi.org/10.1177/0093854808327277.

Chapter 10:

Abbasi, Irum Saeed. "Social Media Addiction in Romantic Relationships: Does User's Age Influence Vulnerability to Social Media Infidelity?" *Personality and Individual Differences* 139 (March 2019): 277–280. https://doi.org/10.1016/j.paid.2018.10.038.

Biino, Marta. "How Much Money OnlyFans Creators Make." *Business Insider*, May 9, 2024. www.businessinsider.com/how-much-money-onlyfans-creators-make-real-examples-2023-1?op=1.

Burtăverde, Vlad, et al. "Why Do People Watch Porn? An Evolutionary Perspective on the Reasons for Pornography Consumption." *Evolutionary Psychology* 19, no. 2 (April 2021). https://doi.org/10.1177/14747049211028798.

de Alarcón, Rubén, Javier I. de la Iglesia, Nerea M. Casado, and Angel L. Montejo. "Online Porn Addiction: What We Know and What We Don't—A Systematic Review." *Journal of Clinical Medicine* 8, no. 1 (January 2019): 91. https://pmc.ncbi.nlm.nih.gov/articles/PMC6352245/.

Emamzadeh, Arash. "New Research: 8 Common Reasons People Use Porn." *Psychology Today*, May 9, 2021. www.psychologytoday.com/us/blog/finding-new-home/202105/new-research-8-common-reasons-people-use-porn.

Giroux, Caroline. "Early Exposure to Pornography: A Form of Sexual Trauma." *Journal of Psychiatry Reform* 10, no. 15 (December 2021).

Grubbs, Joshua B., et al. "Self-Reported Addiction to Pornography in a Nationally Representative Sample: The Roles of Use Habits, Religiousness, and Moral Incongruence." *Journal of Behavioral Addictions* 8, no. 1 (January 2019): 88–93. https://doi.org/10.1556/2006.7.2018.134.

Levine, Beth. "Does Using Porn Lead to Erectile Dysfunction?" *EverydayHealth.com*, July 22, 2020. www.everydayhealth.com/erectile-dysfunction/pornography-habit-is-linked-to-erectile-dysfunction-research-suggests/.

Ley, David J. *Ethical Porn for Dicks: A Man's Guide to Responsible Viewing Pleasure*. Stone Bridge Press, 2016.

Lippmann, Marie, et al. "Learning on OnlyFans: User Perspectives on Knowledge and Skills Acquired on the Platform." *Sexuality & Culture* 27, no. 4 (January 2023): 1203–1223. https://doi.org/10.1007/s12119-022-10060-0.

Litam, Stacey Diane, et al. "Sexual Attitudes and Characteristics of OnlyFans Users." *Archives of Sexual Behavior* 51, no. 6 (July 2022): 3093–3103. https://doi.org/10.1007/s10508-022-02329-0.

McKee, Alan, et al. "The Criteria to Identify Pornography that can Support Healthy Sexual Development for Young Adults: Results of an International Delphi Panel." *International Journal of Sexual Health* 35, no. 1 (January 2023): 1–12. https://doi.org/10.1080/19317611.2022.2161030.

Mestre-Bach, Gemma, et al. "Pornography Use and Violence: A Systematic Review of the Last 20 Years." *Trauma, Violence & Abuse* 25, no. 2 (June 2023): 1088–1112. https://doi.org/10.1177/15248380231173619.

Newstrom, Nicholas P., and Steven M. Harris. "Pornography and Couples: What Does the Research Tell Us?" *Contemporary Family Therapy* 38, no. 4 (December 2016). https://www.researchgate.net/publication/307620661_Pornography_and_Couples_What_Does_the_Research_Tell_Us.

Park, J. I., et al. "The Differentiation Between Consumers of Hentai Pornography and Human Pornography." *Sexologies* 31, no. 3 (September 2022): 226–239. https://doi.org/10.1016/j.sexol.2021.11.002.

Perry, Samuel L., and Cyrus Schleifer. "Till Porn Do Us Part? A Longitudinal Examination of Pornography Use and Divorce." *Journal of Sex Research* 55, no. 3 (May 2017): 284–296. https://doi.org/10.1080/00224499.2017.1317709.

Peter, Jochen, and Patti M. Valkenburg. "Adolescents and Pornography: A Review of 20 Years of Research." *Journal of Sex Research* 53, no. 4–5 (March 2016): 509–531. https://doi.org/10.1080/00224499.2016.1143441.

Statista Research Department. "OnlyFans - Statistics & Facts." *Statista*, July 2, 2024. www.statista.com/topics/10083/onlyfans/.

Steele, Vaughn R., et al. "Sexual Desire, Not Hypersexuality, Is Related to Neurophysiological Responses Elicited by Sexual Images." *Socioaffective Neuroscience & Psychology* 3, no. 1 (January 2013): 20770. https://doi.org/10.3402/snp.v3i0.20770.

Szymanski, Dawn M., et al. "Sexual Minority Women's Relationship Quality: Examining the Roles of Multiple Oppressions and Silencing the Self." *Psychology of Sexual Orientation and Gender Diversity* 3, no. 1 (March 2016): 1–10. https://doi.org/10.1037/sgd0000145.

Chapter 11:

Amos, Natalie, and Marita McCabe. "Positive Perceptions of Genital Appearance and Feeling Sexually Attractive: Is It a Matter of Sexual Esteem?" *Archives of Sexual Behavior* 45, no. 5 (July 2016): 1249–1258. https://pubmed.ncbi.nlm.nih.gov/26857376/.

Associated Press. "About 333,000 Children Were Abused within France's Catholic Church, a Report Finds." *NPR*, October 5, 2021. www.npr.org/2021/10/05/1043302348/france-catholic-church-sexual-abuse-report-children.

Beaulieu, Noémie, et al. "Toward an Integrative Model of Intimacy, Sexual Satisfaction, and Relationship Satisfaction: A Prospective Study in Long-Term Couples." *Journal of Sex Research* 60, no. 8 (October 2022): 1100–1112. https://doi.org/10.1080/00224499.2022.2129557.

Cross, Katie. "'I Have the Power in My Body to Make People Sin': The Trauma of Purity Culture and the Concept of 'Body Theodicy.'" In *Feminist Trauma Theologies: Body, Scripture and Church in Critical Perspective*, edited by K. O'Donnell and K. Cross. SCM Press, 2020.

Ford, Brett Q., et al. "The Psychological Health Benefits of Accepting Negative Emotions and Thoughts: Laboratory, Diary, and Longitudinal Evidence."

Journal of Personality and Social Psychology 115, no. 6 (July 2017): 1075–1092. https://doi.org/10.1037/pspp0000157.

Fry, Richard. "Women Now Outnumber Men in the U.S. College-Educated Labor Force." Pew Research Center, September 26, 2022. https://www.pewresearch.org/short-reads/2022/09/26/women-now-outnumber-men-in-the-u-s-college-educated-labor-force/.

García-Sancho, E., et al. "Relationship Between Emotional Intelligence and Aggression: A Systematic Review." *Aggression and Violent Behavior* 19, no. 5 (September 2014): 584–591. https://doi.org/10.1016/j.avb.2014.07.007.

Gaunt, Ruth. "Breadwinners vs. Caregivers: Why Outdated Family Roles Are Bad for Everyone." In *Essays on Equality: The Politics of Childcare*, edited by Becca Shepard and George May. King's College London, 2023.

Gish, Elizabeth. "'Are You a "Trashable" Styrofoam Cup?': Harm and Damage Rhetoric in the Contemporary American Sexual Purity Movement." *Journal of Feminist Studies in Religion* 34, no. 2 (2018): 5. https://doi.org/10.2979/jfemistudreli.34.2.03.

Griffin, K. R. "An Examination of the Association of Religiosity, Purity Culture, and Religious Trauma with Symptoms of Depression and Anxiety." PhD diss., University of Nevada, Las Vegas, 2023.

Jafarian, T., M. Fathi, M. Arshi, and R. Ghaderi. "The Effect of Men's Emotional Intelligence on Violence Against Women Among Married Couples." *Knowledge & Research in Applied Psychology* 16, no. 4 (2017): 76–83.

Jones, Alyssa C., and Jordyn M. Tipsword, et al. "Fear of Sin and Fear of God: Scrupulosity Predicts Women's Daily Experiences of Mental Contamination Following Sexual Trauma." *Journal of Traumatic Stress* 36, no. 5 (August 2023): 932–942. https://doi.org/10.1002/jts.22961.

Kohler, Hans-Peter, et al. "Partner + Children = Happiness? The Effects of Partnerships and Fertility on Well-Being." *Population and Development Review* 31, no. 3 (October 2005): 407–445. https://doi.org/10.1111/j.1728-4457.2005.00078.x.

Korhonen, Veera. "U.S. Approval of Interracial Marriage by Age Group 2021." *Statista*, July 5, 2024. www.statista.com/statistics/1405681/us-approval-of-interracial-marriage-by-age-group/.

Lever, Janet, et al. "Does Size Matter? Men's and Women's Views on Penis Size Across the Lifespan." *Psychology of Men & Masculinity* 7, no. 3 (July 2006): 129–143. https://doi.org/10.1037/1524-9220.7.3.129.

Matud, M. Pilar. "Masculine/Instrumental and Feminine/Expressive Traits and Health, Well-Being, and Psychological Distress in Spanish Men." *American Journal of Men's Health* 13, no. 1 (February 2019). https://doi.org/10.1177/1557988319832749.

Mitchell, Travis. "1. Trends and Patterns in Intermarriage." Pew Research Center, May 18, 2017. www.pewresearch.org/social-trends/2017/05/18/1-trends-and-patterns-in-intermarriage/.

Rice, Simon, et al. "Gender Norms and the Mental Health of Boys and Young Men." *Lancet Public Health* 6, no. 8 (August 2021): 541–542. https://doi.org/10.1016/s2468-2667(21)00138-9.

Singh, Devendra. "Female Judgment of Male Attractiveness and Desirability for Relationships: Role of Waist-to-Hip Ratio and Financial Status." *Journal of Personality and Social Psychology* 69, no. 6 (1995): 1089–1101. https://doi.org/10.1037//0022-3514.69.6.1089.

Stillwell, Amelia, and Brian S. Lowery. "Gendered Racial Boundary Maintenance: Social Penalties for White Women in Interracial Relationships." *Journal of Personality and Social Psychology* 121, no. 3 (September 2021): 548–572. https://doi.org/10.1037/pspi0000332.

Treece, Kiah. "Average Wedding Cost: How Much Should You Budget for Your Big Day?" *Forbes Magazine*, April 3, 2024. www.forbes.com/advisor/personal-loans/average-cost-of-a-wedding/.

Williams, D. J., et al. "'It's Absolutely Intense, and I love It!' A Qualitative Investigation of 'Pegging' as Leisure." *Leisure Sciences* (June 2023): 1–15. https://doi.org/10.1080/01490400.2023.2226669.

Williams, D. J., and Lynnette Coto. "'Best Sex He'd Ever Had!': A Qualitative Analysis of 'Most Amazing' Pegging Experiences." *Journal of Positive Sexuality* 9, no. 2 (December 2023): 15–18. https://doi.org/10.51681/1.923.

Chapter 12:

Banissy, Michael. *Touch Matters: Handshakes, Hugs, and the New Science on How Touch Can Enhance Your Well-Being*. Chronicle Prism, 2023.

Goldmeier, David, and Ali Mears. "Meditation: A Review of Its Use in Western Medicine and, in Particular, Its Role in the Management of Sexual Dysfunction." *Current Psychiatry Reviews* 6, no. 1 (February 2010): 11–14. https://doi.org/10.2174/157340010790596508.

Grewen, Karen M., et al. "Warm Partner Contact is Related to Lower Cardiovascular Reactivity." *Behavioral Medicine* 29, no. 3 (January 2003): 123–130. https://doi.org/10.1080/08964280309596065.

Kim, Jean H., et al. "Sociodemographic Correlates of Sexlessness Among American Adults and Associations with Self-Reported Happiness Levels: Evidence from the U.S. General Social Survey." *Archives of Sexual Behavior* 46, no. 8 (March 2017): 2403–2415. https://doi.org/10.1007/s10508-017-0968-7.

Kimmes, Jonathan G., et al. "A Treatment Model for Anxiety-Related Sexual Dysfunctions Using Mindfulness Meditation within a Sex-Positive Framework." *Sexual and Relationship Therapy* 30, no. 2 (February 2015): 286–296. https://doi.org/10.1080/14681994.2015.1013023.

Konda, Mayuresh Vasudevan. "Social Touch: Investigating the Effect of Mediated Social Touch on Social Presence." Master's thesis, University of Twente, 2022. https://essay.utwente.nl/92190/1/Konda_MA_EEMCS.pdf.

McCreary, Simone L., and Kevin G. Alderson. "The Perceived Effects of Practicing Meditation on Women's Sexual and Relational Lives." *Sexual and Relationship Therapy* 28, no. 1–2 (February 2013): 105–119. https://doi.org/10.1080/14681994.2013.770830.

Rea, Shilo. "Hugs Help Protect against Stress and Infection, Say Carnegie Mellon Researchers." Carnegie Mellon University, December 17, 2014. www.cmu.edu/news/stories/archives/2014/december/december17_hugsprotect.html.

Suvilehto, Juulia T., et al. "Topography of Social Touching Depends on Emotional Bonds Between Humans." *Proceedings of the National Academy of Sciences* 112, no. 45 (October 2015): 13811–13816. https://doi.org/10.1073/pnas.1519231112.

Chapter 13:

Alarie, Milaine. "Family and Consensual Non-monogamy: Parents' Perceptions of Benefits and Challenges." *Journal of Marriage and Family* 86, no. 2 (December 2023): 494–512. https://doi.org/10.1111/jomf.12955.

Bergstrand, Curtis, and Jennifer Blevins Williams. "Today's Alternative Marriage Styles: The Case of Swingers." *Journal of Human Sexuality* 3 (October 2000).

Carlson, Daniel L., et al. "The Gendered Division of Housework and Couples' Sexual Relationships: A Reexamination." *Journal of Marriage and Family* 78, no. 4 (May 2016): 975–995. https://doi.org/10.1111/jomf.12313.

Conley, Terri D., et al. "Sexual Satisfaction Among Individuals in Monogamous and Consensually Non-monogamous Relationships." *Journal of Social and Personal Relationships* 35, no. 4 (March 2018): 509–531. https://doi.org/10.1177/0265407517743078.

Daminger, Allison. "De-gendered Processes, Gendered Outcomes: How Egalitarian Couples Make Sense of Non-egalitarian Household Practices." *American Sociological Review* 85, no. 5 (September 2020): 806–829. https://doi.org/10.1177/0003122420950208.

Fairbrother, Nichole, et al. "Open Relationship Prevalence, Characteristics, and Correlates in a Nationally Representative Sample of Canadian Adults." *Journal of Sex Research* 56, no. 6 (April 2019): 695–704. https://doi.org/10.1080/00224499.2019.1580667.

Fleckenstein, James R., and Derrell W. Cox. "The Association of an Open Relationship Orientation with Health and Happiness in a Sample of Older US Adults." *Sexual and Relationship Therapy* 30, no. 1 (November 2014): 94–116. https://doi.org/10.1080/14681994.2014.976997.

Fry, Richard, et al. "In a Growing Share of U.S. Marriages, Husbands and Wives Earn about the Same." Pew Research Center, April 13, 2023. www.pewresearch.org/social-trends/2023/04/13/in-a-growing-share-of-u-s-marriages-husbands-and-wives-earn-about-the-same/.

Guy-Evans, Olivia. "Ethical Non-Monogamy: Basics & Rules for ENM Relationships." *Simply Psychology*, January 18, 2024. www.simplypsychology.org/what-is-ethical-non-monogamy.html.

Kinsey Institute. "Polyamory and Consensual Non-Monogamy in the US." Kinsey Institute Research Institute News, June 17, 2022. blogs.iu.edu/kinseyinstitute/2022/06/17/polyamory-and-consensual-non-monogamy-in-the-us/.

Klug, Hope. "Why Monogamy? A Review of Potential Ultimate Drivers." *Frontiers in Ecology and Evolution* 6 (March 2018). https://doi.org/10.3389/fevo.2018.00030.

Mallenbaum, Carly, and Mimi Montgomery. "Polyamory Gets More Attention and Legal Protection." *Axios*, February 15, 2024. www.axios.com/2024/02/14/polyamory-laws-nonmonogamy-stigma.

Matsick, Jes L., et al. "Love and Sex: Polyamorous Relationships Are Perceived More Favorably than Swinging and Open Relationships." *Psychology & Sexuality* 5, no. 4 (September 2013): 339–348. https://doi.org/10.1080/19419899.2013.832934.

Mogilski, Justin K., et al. "Monogamy versus Consensual Non-monogamy: Alternative Approaches to Pursuing a Strategically Pluralistic Mating Strategy." *Archives of*

Sexual Behavior 46, no. 2 (December 2015): 407–417. https://doi.org/10.1007/s10508-015-0658-2.

"Monogamy Definition & Meaning." *Merriam-Webster*. www.merriam-webster.com/dictionary/monogamy.

Moors, Amy C., Amanda N. Gesselman, et al. "Desire, Familiarity, and Engagement in Polyamory: Results from a National Sample of Single Adults in the United States." *Frontiers in Psychology* 12 (March 2021). https://doi.org/10.3389/fpsyg.2021.619640.

Moors, Amy C., et al. "Unique and Shared Relationship Benefits of Consensually Non-monogamous and Monogamous Relationships." *European Psychologist* 22, no. 1 (January 2017): 55–71. https://doi.org/10.1027/1016-9040/a000278.

Savage, Dan. "Monogamish." Savage Love, *Chicago Reader*, July 21, 2011. https://chicagoreader.com/columns-opinion/savage-love-monogamish/.

Wentworth, Diane Keyser, and Robert M. Chell. "The Role of Househusband and Housewife as Perceived by a College Population." *Journal of Psychology* 135, no. 6 (November 2001): 639–650. https://doi.org/10.1080/00223980109603725.

Resource Library

Chapter 2:

Bass, Ellen, and Laura Davis. *The Courage to Heal: A Guide for Women Survivors of Child Sexual Abuse*. The Courage to Heal Press, 2015.

Carnagey, Melissa Pintor. *Sex Positive Talks to Have with Kids: A Guide to Raising Sexually Healthy, Informed, Empowered Young People*. Sex Positive Families, 2020.

Davis, Tchiki. "A Guide to Affirmations and How to Use Them." *Psychology Today*, Sussex Publishers, www.psychologytoday.com/us/blog/click-here-for-happiness/202105/a-guide-to-affirmations-and-how-to-use-them.

Dodson, Betty. *Sex for One: The Joy of Selfloving*. Three Rivers Press, 2012.

Haines, Staci, and Felice Newman. *Healing Sex: A Mind-Body Approach to Healing Sexual Trauma*. Cleis Press, 2007.

Jeglic, Elizabeth L. "How to Cope Following Sexual Abuse." *Psychology Today*, Sussex Publishers, www.psychologytoday.com/us/blog/protecting-children-sexual-abuse/202109/how-cope-following-sexual-abuse. Accessed 3 Sept. 2024.

Labanz, Julie. "Boost Your Sexual Confidence." *Psychology Today*, Sussex Publishers, https://www.psychologytoday.com/us/blog/sexual-self-discovery/202406/boost-your-sexual-confidence.

Levine, Peter A. *Healing Trauma: A Pioneering Program for Restoring the Wisdom of the Body*. Sounds True, 2008.

Rothschild, Babette. *8 Keys to Safe Trauma Recovery: Take-Charge Strategies to Empower Your Healing*. W.W. Norton & Co, 2012.

Suwinyattichaiporn, Tara. "What's Your Sexual Profile?" *Luvbites by Dr. Tara*, www.luvbites.co/quizzes/whats-your-sexual-profile.

Van der Kolk, Bessel A. *The Body Keeps the Score: Brain, Mind, and Body in the Healing of Trauma*. Blackstone, 2014.

Chapter 6:

Brotto, Lori A., Emily Nagoski, et al. *Better Sex through Mindfulness: How Women Can Cultivate Desire*. Greystone Books, 2018.

Harris, Stella. *Tongue Tied: Untangling Communication in Sex, Kink, and Relationships*. Cleis Press, 2018.

Nelson, Tammy. *Getting the Sex You Want: Shed Your Inhibitions and Reach New Heights of Passion Together*. Quiver, 2013.

Wise, Nan J. "How to Talk about Sex with Your Partner." *Psychology Today*, Sussex Publishers, https://www.psychologytoday.com/us/blog/why-good-sex-matters/202204/how-talk-about-sex-your-partner.